Manual of
SKIN DISEASES

By the same author (Anil Dashore)

MCQ's in Dermatology Venerology and Leprology

Manual of Skin Diseases

VIJAY K. JAIN M.D.
Consultant Dermatologist
Department of Skin, V.D. and Leprosy
Medical College and Hospital
ROHTAK (Haryana)

ANIL DASHORE
Consultant Dermatologist
Choithram Hospital & Research Centre
INDORE (M.P)

CBS

CBS PUBLISHERS & DISTRIBUTORS PVT. LTD.
New Delhi • Bangalore • Pune • Cochin • Chennai (India)

ISBN : 81-239-0966-7

First Edition : 1994
Reprint : 1996, 1998, 2000, 2003,
2005, 2007, 2010, 2013

Published by Satish Kumar Jain and produced by V.K. Jain for
CBS Publishers & Distributors Pvt. Ltd.,
CBS Plaza, 4819/XI Prahlad Street, 24 Ansari Road, Daryaganj,
New Delhi - 110002, India. • Website: www.cbspd.com
e-mail: delhi@cbspd.com, cbspubs@airtelmail.in
Ph.: 23289259, 23266861, 23266867 • Fax: 011-23243014

Branches:

- ***Bengaluru:*** Seema House, 2975, 17th Cross, K.R. Road, Bansankari 2nd Stage, Bengaluru - 560070
  • Ph.: +91-80-26771678/79 • Fax: +91-80-26771680
  • E-mail: cbsbng@gmail.com, bangalore@cbspd.com
- ***Pune:*** Bhuruk Prestige, Sr. No. 52/12/2+1+3/2, Narhe, Haveli (Near Katraj-Dehu Road By-pass), Pune - 411041
  • Ph.: +91-20-64704058/59, 32342277 • E-mail: pune@cbspd.com
- ***Kochi:*** 36/14, Kalluvilakam, Lissie Hospital Road, Kochi - 682018, Kerala • Ph.: +91-484-4059061-65
  • Fax: +91-484-4059065 • E-mail: cochin@cbspd.com
- ***Chennai:*** 20, West Park Road, Shenoy Nagar, Chennai - 600030
  Ph.: +91-44-26260666, 26208620 • Fax: +91-44-42032115
  • E-mail: chennai@cbspd.com

Printed at :
J.S. Offset Printers, Delhi

Preface

We have tried to compress the universe of skin diseases in this small booklet. All through the book, we, especially kept in mnid the mddical students and general practitioners other than the dermatologists for whom the word of dermatology is an alien one. With this in mind every effort has been made to present the subject in a comprehensive and lucid manner. The text also includes colour plates and black and white pictures for the purposes of illustration.

We are grateful to Dr. D.R. Arora, Assoc. Professor (Microbiology) for his esteemed contribution to the chapter on AIDS.

We should like to thank Mr. Ravinder Mr. J.K. Sarin for photgraphic assistance and Mr. V.P. Grover for assistance in drawing the diagrams.

We are deeply indebted to Shri Satish Kumar Jain (CBS Publishers & Ditributors) for their keen interest and devotion in getting this book published. Credit goes to Shri Vinod Kumar Jain for giving the present get-up to the book. We are also thankful to Shri Anil Kumar (Maharani Printers) for prompt printing and release of the book.

We also owe an incalculable debt to our families who were willing to share with us this endeavor.

ANIL DASHORE
V.K. JAIN

Contents

1

Anatomy, Physiology and Pathology

ANATOMY

The skin forms a self replacing, multifunctional covering over the surface of the body which isolates it from the environment. It is the largest organ of the body which amounts to about 15% of the body weight.

The skin is composed of three layers: the epidermis, the dermis and the subcutaneous tissue.

The appendages of the skin are the hair, the nails, the sebaeceus glands and the sweet glands. In addition, this complicated structure is supplied with two horizontal and parallel plexuses of blood vessels; two corresponding sets of lymphatic vessels; and two similarly distributed supplies of nerve tissues consisting of medulated and nonmedulated fibres.

Epidermis

The epidermis contains no blood vessels of its own and is dependent on the vascular and tissue fluid supply of the dermis for its sustenance. Microscopic examination reveals that the epidermis is clearly separable into four areas:

1. Basal cell layer (Stratum germinosum)
2. Prickle cell layer (Stratum malpighii)
3. Granular cell layer (Stratum granulosum)
4. Horny cell layer (Stratum corneum)

These represent transitional stages in the keratinization of the epidermal cells as it moves towards the surface.

1. *Basal Cell Layer (Stratum Germinosum)*

The deepest of the epidermal layers, adjacent to the dermis, is the basal cell layer. It consists of a single row of columnar cells arranged vertically to the basement membrane and with a centrally placed nucleus. Melanocytes are seen in basal layer on electron microscopy.

2. *Prickle Cell Layer (Stratum Malpighii)*

The prickle cell layer lies upon the basal layer and occupies most of the epidermis. It is made up of polygonal cells that become flatten as they migrate towards the surface. These cells are joined to each other by multiple protrusions from each cell that appear on examination by light microscope and in routine staining as intercellular bridges or 'Prickles'. Electron microscopy has demonstrated that adjacent cells have, at their point of contact, areas of thickened membranes called desosomes. If Gold stain is employed one may observe gold impregnated cells with dendritic processes in between prickle cells. These are called Langerhans cells which have no desmosomes and donot possess dopa oxidase activity.

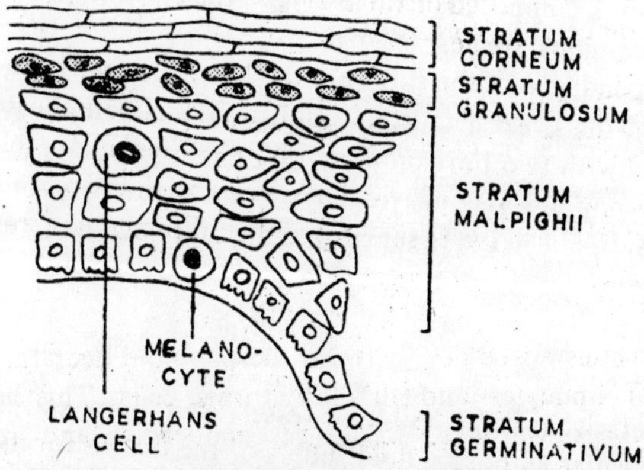

Fig. 1 Vertical section of epiderms in diagrammatic form

3. *Granular Layer (Stratum Granulosum)*

The granular layer cells are one to three row thick and lies on top of prickle cell layer. These cells contain irregular granules of keratohyaline which are deeply basophilic.

4. *Horny Cell Layer (Stratum Corneum)*

It consists of several rows of flattened, completely cornified horn cells without nucleus. The surface row of the cells appears as thin, dry scales. This layer is the thickest on the palms of the hands and the soles of the feet and thinnest on the eyelids and the prepuce. The stratum lucidum consists of a thin strip of glistening, translucent, flattened cells without granules, occasionally seen between stratum corneum and granular layer especially on palms and soles.

Dermis

The dermis rests upon a thick pad of subcutaneous fat. It is about 10-30 times thicker than epidermis. It consists of collagen, elastic fibres and ground substance within which blood vessels, lymph vessels, nerves, pilosebaceous, apocrine and eccrine sweat units are embedded. The dermis may be divided into two compartments:

(a) *Papillary Dermis*

A thin zone which lies immediately beneath the epidermis composed of thin haphazardly arranged collagen fibres, fibroblasts, abundant ground substance and blood vessels.

(b) *Reticular Dermis*

A thick zone consisting of dense collagen and elastic fibres lies in between papillary dermis and subcutaneous fat. It contains less fibroblast, blood vessels and ground substance than papillary dermis.

Subcutaneous Tissue

The subcutaneous tissue lies between dermis and deep fascia and is composed of lipocytes and the fat storage cells. This sheet of fat varies in thickness with age, sex, race, endocrinal and nutritional status of the subject. It protects the body from trauma and cold.

PHYSIOLOGY

Functions of the Skin

1. Skin acts as a natural covering of the body and protects the underlying structures, especially in relation to maintenance of the body equilibrium against the destructive effects of the environment.

2. It plays an important part in regulation of body temperature.
3. It maintains itself and repairs its own wounds quickly and efficiently by two distinct epidermal and dermal processes.
4. It participates in the production of vitamin-D.
5. It supports a continuously operating chemical factory of carbohydrate, protein, fat and androgen metabolism.
6. It produces secretions from its sebaceous and eccrine surface glands that maintain a buffered protective film.
7. It helps in elimination of waste products through perspiration.
8. It operates its own delayed hypersensitivity mechanism and devlops an immune reaction from simple contact with foreign materials as soon as they have been identified as such. It acts as a sense organ. The specialized receptors of the skin receive various stimuli from the external environment and transmit the stimulation of central nervous system.

PATHOLOGY

The common pathological terms used in dermatology are:

Hyperkeratosis

Increased thickening of stratum corneum.

Parakeratosis

Presence of immature nucleated cells in the stratum corneum.

Dyskeratosis

Premature keratinization of individual epidermal cells.

Acanthosis

Increase in thickness of prickle cell layer due to stimulation of basal layer.

Atrophy

Consists of thinning of all the layers of the epidermis and is accompanied by flattening of the papillae.

Acantholysis

The loss of coherence between epidermal or epithelial cells.

Spongiosis (Intercellular oedema)

Accumulation of fluid between the epidermal cells.

Hydropic Degeneration of Basal cells

A type of degeneration causing vacuolization of basal cells.

Caseation Necrosis

Necrosis associated with formation of caseation, a pale eosinophilic, amorphous, finely granular material.

Granuloma

A chronic proliferative lesion, consisting of mononuclear cells and either epithelioid cells or multinucleated giant cell or both.

Langhans Giant Cell

A large multinucleated cell formed by collection of epitheloid cells. The arrangement of nuclei are in a horseshoe pattern.

Grenz Zone

A narrow clear zone that may be found between the epidermis and dermal lesion.

Foam Cell

Macrophage with foamy appearance containing high proportion of dead lepra-bacilli.

TYPES OF SKIN LESIONS

The morphology of skin lesion is the essential element for the clinical diagnosis of the disease. There is difference in opinion about the size and depth of the lesions.

The lesions fall in three types:

Flat Lesions

These lesions are neither raised from surface nor depress from the surface. These are:

Macule

It is a flat, circumscribed discolouration of the skin and mucus membrane without change in texture upto 1 cm in its longest diameter. It may be hyperpigmented, hypopigmented, depigmented or erythematous.

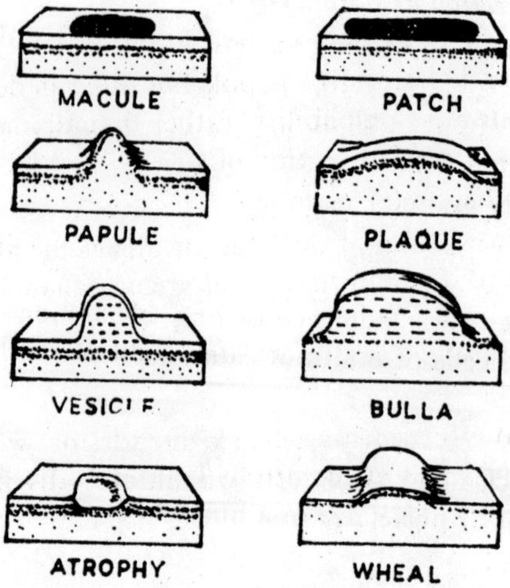

Fig. 2 Skin lesions: Morphology

Patch

Macule larger than 1 cm is described as patch or area.

Purpura

It is exavasations of RBC in the skin. On application of pressure with a glass slide redness will not disappear. Small, pinpoint purpuric spots are known as *Petechiae* and large, bruiselike purpuric spots are known as *Ecchymoses*.

Telangiectasia

They are permanent dilatations of capillaries that may or may not disappear with application of pressure.

Elevated Lesions

Papule

A solid, elevated lesion of the skin or mucus membrane upto 1 cm in its longest diameter. Papules may have variety of shapes and colour.

Plaque

It is a flat solid lesion elevated above the surface of adjoining skin, with horizontal dimensions much more than the vertical ones.

Nodule

It is a solid, palpable lesion like papule but differ in depth of involvement and/or substantive palpability, rather than diameter.

Tumour

It is a solid elevated lesion of the skin or mucus membrane with the added dimension of depth in tissue and greater than 1 cm its longest diameter.

Wheal

A wheal is that topped oedematous, elevated lesion with sharply demarked margins which is evanescent in nature, disappearing within hours.

Vesicle

A vesicle is circumscribed, elevated clear fluid containing lesion which have size of 0.5 cm diameter.

Bullae

A bulla is a large vesicle having diameter greater than 0.5 cm.

Pustule

It is same as vesicle but it contains purulent exudate instead of clear fluid.

Abscess

It is a localized accumulation of purulent material deep in dermis or subcutaneous tissue.

Scale

Scale is an abnormal shedding of stratum corneum because of rapid keratinization.

Crust

Crust is a layer of dried-up secretions (serum, blood or purulent exudate).

Lichenification

Lichenified areas refer to thickened plaques with accentuated skin markings.

Depressed Lesions

Erosion

It is a superficial break in continuty of skin which involves epidermal portion only.

Ulcer

In this type of the lesions, break in continuity of skin involving epidermis and at least upper part of dermis.

Atrophy

It means thinning of the layers of the skin.

Scar

Scar is a proliferation of collagen tissue formed during healing process of any discontinuity.

Sclerosis

Sclerosis means localized or diffuse thickening or induration in the skin.

2

Topical Therapy

The general principles of dermatological therapy differ in no way from those of any other branch of medicine. Dermatologist have an added advantage of selecting a topical route of administration of drugs. The topical therapy is the easiest and often the most important mode of treatment.

Main actions of topical therapy are soothing and drying effect, hydration of stratum corneum in dry conditions, and removal of debris thus bringing the drug directly to the target organ and avoiding the multiorgan exposure of drug as seen in systemic administration.

Topical therapy has two major components, the medicinal ingredient and the vehicle or base by which the medicine is carried to the skin. The different agents used in topical therapy are available as liquids, compresses, soaks and bath (Wetdressings lotions), or as solids (powders, creams or ointments). Liquids are the most useful for acute exudative lesions while creams and ointments are usually given for deeper or more chronic lesions.

Liquids

The active ingredient of compresses, soaks and baths is water. The various medicaments may be added to the water. These include potassium permanganate, aluminium acetate (Burrows solution), common salt, liquor piscis carbonis and silver nitrate.

Lotions may be clear (potassium permanganate, castellanis paint, tincture of iodine) or shake lotions (calamine). Shake lotions are suspensions of powders in liquid base.

Solids

Creams are of two types i.e. cold cream (water in oil emulsion) and vanishing cream (oil in water emulsion). Both the creams can be used as basis for other medicament. Creams are easy to apply and lead to an effective penetration of the medication.

Ointments are suspensions of an active ingredient in an oily vehicle. Common vehicles are petrolatum and paraffin. These vehicles keep the active agents in contact with skin for a long period.

Powders are helpful in intertriginous areas. They promote drying effect by increasing evaporation of water from skin surfaces.

Commonly used topical preparations are:

Anti-inflammatory Agents

Topical corticosteroids are the most potent antiinflammatory preparations. These can be of the two types, fluorinated or nonfluorinated. Fluorinated steroids (fluocinolone acetonide) are more effective and generally used for actively inflammed lesions. Continuous long term applications may lead to atrophy, striae and telangiectasia. The non-fluorinated steroids (hydrocortisone) are least potent, slower to act and may be used over a long period.

Antibacterial Agents

Antibacterial agents are frequently used for skin infections. The common antibacterial agents are gentian violet (1%), brilliant green (1%), tincture iodine, povidone iodine (10%), silver nitrate (1-2%), polymyxin B, neomycin, clindamycin, gentamycin, erythromycin and sodium fusidate.

Keratolytic Agents

These agents are used to dissolve or remove the thickened stratum corneum. Salicylic acid (3-10%), urea (10-20%) and resorcinol (1%), are often used as keratolytic agents.

Antipruritic Agents

The common antipruritic agents are phenol (1-2%), menthol (0.1-1%). camphor (2-5%), calamine and crotomiton (10%) lotion.

Antifungal Agents

Miconazole (2%), clotrimazole (1%), econazole (1%), tolnaftate (1%). nystatin, haymycin and ciclopirox olamine (1%) can be used locally as antifungal agents.

Antiparasitic Agents

Crotomiton (10%), gamma benzene hexachloride (1%), benzyl benzoate emulsion (25%) and sulphur (5-10%) are useful in various types of parasitosis.

Sunscreens

The agents which protect the skin from sunlight are paraaminobenzoic acid (5-10%), titanium dioxide (10%), zinc oxide (10%), and benzophenones (5-10%).

Antiviral Agents

The common antiviral agents are idoxuridine, acylovir and vidarabine.

Caustics

Caustics are the destructive agents useful in treatment of warts, xanthelasma and hyperplastic lesions. The commonly used caustics are trichloroacetic acid (50-100%), phenol (80%) and silver nitrate (10-20%).

3

Bacterial Diseases

The bacterial flora of normal skin is of two types: (a) transient: which get on to the skin surface from the environment and (b) resident: which can multiply and are regularly present on the skin. The common resident organisms are staphylococcus, corynebacterium acne and the aerobic diphtheroids. Various types of bacterial infections of the skin are:

(A) Extra Follicular Infections (Involvement of Extra Follicular Portions of the Skin)

(a) *Superficial*:

—*Impetigo Contagiosa*
—Bullous impetigo
—Staphylococcal scalded skin syndrome.

(b) *Deep*:

—*Ecthyma*
—Erysipelas
—Cellulitis

(B) Follicular Infections (Involves Hair Follicles)

(a) *Superficiul—Follicular Impetigo of Bockhart*

(b) *Deep*:

—*Sycosis*
—Furunculosis
—Carbuncle

IMPETIGO CONTAGIOSA

It is a contagious superficial infection of the skin commonly due to streptococci or mixed infection. Predisposing factors are poor hygiene, high humidity and infection from existing skin conditions such as pediculosis, scabies or eczemas. It is more common in children than adults.

Impetigo starts as a thin walled vesicle on an erythematous background which soon turns into pustule. Vesicles and pustules rupture readily and produce 'stuck on' dirty yellow crusts. Removal of crusts reveal a red weeping surface. Gradual extension of the lesion occur with or without central healing. New satellite lesions may appear. The individual lesion rarely exceed 1 to 2 cm, but occasionally multiple lesions through coalescence may form large lesions. The lesions are superficially located and heal without scarring or atrophy. The face, especially around the nose and mouth, and the limbs are the most commonly affected sites. Regional adenitis with fever may be present in severe cases. Disease tends to clear up spontaneously within 2-3 weeks.

BULLOUS IMPETIGO

This is staphylococcal infection of the skin which manifests as a superficial thin roofed bulla which lasts for 2-3 days before rupturing to produce a mild brownish crusted raw area which heals in the centre and extend peripherally to give rise to circinate lesion. It is predominantly seen in infants but can affect any age. The face is most commonly affected but any area of the body may be involved.

Complications of Impetigo are acute glomerulonephritis, deep cellulitis and bacteriaemia.

Diagnosis

It usually presents no difficulties when the lesions are seen at the stage of crusting. When lesions are circinate, ring worm may be considered in differential diagnosis but here the vesicles are usually small and peripheral and thick crusts are not formed.

Treatment of Impetigo

Crusted lesions must be compressed with potassium permanganate or normal saline solution. Following this, an antibacterial agent should be applied on the lesions. One per cent gentian violet or brilliant green are quite effective antibacterial dyes. Antibiotic ointment such as tetracycline, neomycin, fucidin, gentamycin, soframycin etc. can be applied topically. When the condition is extensive, systemic antibiotic should be given to avoid complications.

STAPHYLOCOCCAL SCALDED SKIN SYNDROME

This is characterised by generalized bullae formation and widespread separation of superficial epidermis from its deeper parts, exposing a moist bright red surface. It is induced by exotoxins produced by group II staphylococcus aureus. Onset is usually preceded by staphylococcal infection elsewhere in the body. It usually occurs in neonates and children. Disease can be fatal and thus requires immediate appropriate antibiotics (Cloxacillin) and fluid therapy.

ECTHYMA

This is essentially a deep form of impetigo surmounted by a firmly adherent often haemorrhagic crust which heals with a scar. Removal of crust reveals a punched out ulcer. Group A stretpococci often initiate the disease. It is most commonly seen on the buttocks, the thighs and the legs and is particularly frequent in individuals with poor nutrition and poor hygiene.

Treatment

It is same as in impetigo. Penicilline, erythromycin or cloxacillin should be given in conjunction with the local treatment. A general assessment of the physical state of the patient should be undertaken.

ERYSIPELAS AND CELLULITIS

Erysipelas is a type of superficial cellulitis in which an oedematous, red, tender, sharply marginated plaque develops which steadily spreads. Fever with rigors may also be associated. The causative organism i.e. β-haemolytic streptococci gain entry to the skin through an ulcer or a crack in the epidermis. It is common on the face, the scalp and the legs

Cellulitis is similar to erysipelas but it involves deeper portion of dermis and subcutaneous tissue. It manifests as a large area of redness, tenderness and swelling with ill defined edges situated on any part of body. Fever with lymphangitis and lymphadenitis may be associated.

Treatment

Penicillin is the drug of choice and should be given for 5 to 7 days. In recurrent cases, long term penicillin may be used prophylactically.

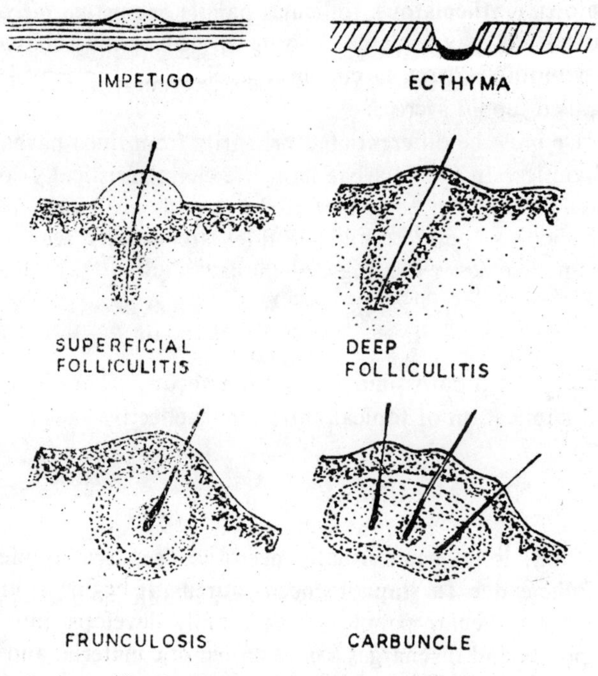

Fig. 3 Diagrammatic representation of pustular lesions

FOLLICULAR IMPETIGO OF BOCKHART

This is a superficial pustular folliculitis usually caused by staphylococcus aureus. The pustules develop in crops and may heal within 7-10 days but sometimes becomes chronic. Common sites are scalp and exterimities. Systemic antibiotic therapy in addition to topical antibiotic ointment is usually necessary though local compresses are equally important.

SYCOSIS BARBAE

Sycosis barbae is chroı , recurrent folliculitis of the beard and moustaches usually due to s.aphylococcus aureus. It is characterized by an oedematous, erythematous, follicular papule or pustule pierced by a hair. The lesions may coalesce to form an oedematous plaque. Lesions heal without scarring. Deep, chronic, cicatracial form of sycosis barbae is called lupoid sycosis.

The disease must be differentiated primarily from tinea barbae and pseudofolliculties. In tinea barbae hair are characteristically loosened or broken off and can be confirmed by mycological examination. In pseudofollicultis, papules and pustules are usually seen on the sides of the neck or over the a·.gle of the jaw.

Treatment

Local treatment with potossium permanganate or warm saline compresses and application of topical antibiotic is effective.

FURUNCLE AND CARBUNCLE

A furuncle (boil) is an acute usually necrotic, deep seated infection of a hair follicle due to staphylococcus aureus. It begins as erythematous, tender follicular papule which rapidly develops into large pustule. It points and discharges a core of necrotic material and heals with a scar. Furuncle occurs commonly on the face, the neck, the axillae and the buttocks. Poor-hygiene, malnutrition, obesity, diabetes, lymphoma and treatment with corticosteroids and cytotoxic drugs are the common predisposing factors.

A carbuncle is a confluent mass of furuncles characterized by painful red, indurated swelling which becomes pustular and necrotic with pus discharging from multiple follicular openings. Moderate to severe constitutional symptoms may be present. It is more common in presence of diabetes, malnutrition and during prolonged corticosteriods therapy. The lesion heals slowly by granulation and scar formation. Common sites are the back, the buttocks and the nape of neck.

Treatment

For milder cases, local compresses with potassium permanganate solution and application of topical antibiotic is effective. A carbuncle or furuncle with surrounding cellulitis must be treated with a systemic antibiotic. Culture and sensitivity test must be performed to determine the antibiotic of choice. In a large, localized fluctuant lesion, incision and drainage is indicated. But too early incision of a furuncle is harmful. Predisposing factors should be corrected to avoid recurrences.

Infections of the skin due to aerobic diptheroids are:

ERYTHRASMA

Erythrasma is a chronic superficial infection of skin, which manifests as asymptomatic, scaly mildly erythematous patches in the axillae, groins and toe webs. It is caused by corynebacterium minutissimum. The organisms produce porphyrins which give coral red fluorescence under wood's light examination. Oral erythromycin 1 gm daily in divided doses for 5-7 days is treatment of choice. Topical antibacterial and keratolytic agents are also effective.

PITTED KERATOLYSIS

Pitted keratolysis is a superficial infection of the skin caused by corynebacterium species manifests as asymptomatic pits on the soles. It responds well to formaline soaks.

TRICHOMYCOSIS AXILLARIS

This is a corynebacterial infection of axillary and pubic hair, characterized by presence of yellow, black or red concretions on the hair shaft. The colour of the sweat may be yellow, black or red according to the colour of the connections. Treatment consists of shaving the hair and topical application of fungicidal ointment or 1-2% aquous formalin.

4

Viral Diseases

There are two main groups of viruses i.e. RNA and DNA viruses. Different viral infections of the skin are commonly caused by DNA group of viruses. These are:

Papilloma virus (warts)

Herpes virus (herpes simplex and herpes zoster)
Pox virus (mollucum contagiosum)

WARTS

Warts are benign, epithelial tumours caused by papilloma group of viruses. These are of five types:

1. Common warts (Verruca vulgaris)
2. Plane warts (Verruca plana)
3. Filiform warts (Verruca filiformis)
4. Plantar warts (Verruca plantaris)
5. Venereal warts (Condyloma acuminata)

Common Warts

These are painless, solid, elevated circumscribed papules or nodules with rough horny projections. They may occur singly or coalesce into larger masses. Isomorphic lesions can be seen at the site of trauma (Koebner phenomenon). A major location of common warts is the dorsum of the hands and feet, wrist, knee, face, nailfolds and underneath the nail. Children are more commonly affected than the adults.

Plane Warts

Plane warts are small, slightly elevated, flat topped, skin coloured papules mostly on the face or hands of children. The number of lesions can vary although they are usually multiple. They are commonly arranged in groups or along a line of trauma (Koebner phenomenon).

Filiform Warts

Filiform warts are small filamentous warts 1-2 mm in length with a cornified tip. They occur most commonly on lips, nostrils, eyelids, axillae and neck. Digitate warts are extensively keratinized and are commonly seen on the scalp.

Plantar Warts

Planter warts occur commonly on the weight bearing parts of the sole and are consequently flat or deep seated. Lesions are rounded, sharply defined with a rough or hyperkeratotic surface. On local pressure lesion is painful. Hyperhidrosis, flat foot and other foot deformities predispose to plantar warts. They may resemble collosities but gentle pairing will reveal a well defined margin, often with fine bleeding point. Mosaic warts result from aggregation of multiple warts which appear as irregular large plaque.

Venereal Warts

They are soft, pink, pedunculated and digitated warts, usually transmitted by sexual contact. High incidence is found in sexually promiscuous young adults. The anogenital region is the most frequently affected site. A moist environment and poor hygiene appear to encourage growth. Massive warts are known as Buschke Lowenstein tumour.

Treatment of Warts

There is no satisfactory treatment of warts. Small warts can be treated with application of 50 to 100%, trichloroacetic acid or phenol. Larger lesions require electrocauterization with currettage or cryotherapy with liquid nitrogen. Topical retinoic acid and 2-4% salicylic acid has been found to be effective in the treatment of plane warts For plantar warts, occlusive dressing of 20-40% salicylic acid is advised for 2-4 days followed by cryotherapy or electrodessication and

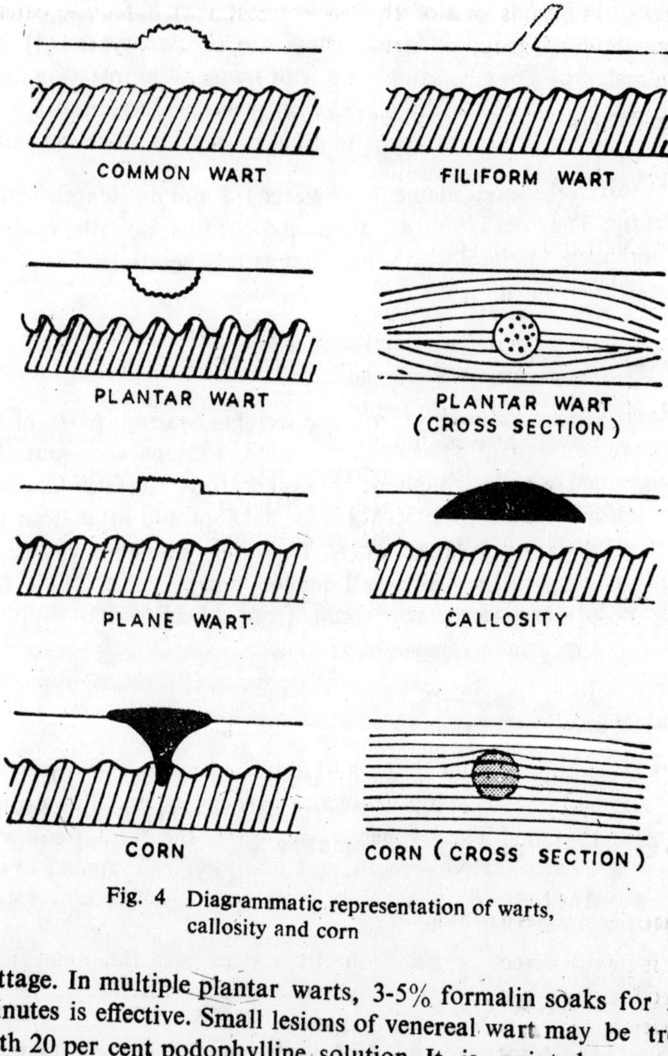

Fig. 4 Diagrammatic representation of warts, callosity and corn

currettage. In multiple plantar warts, 3-5% formalin soaks for 5 to 10 minutes is effective. Small lesions of venereal wart may be treated with 20 per cent podophylline solution. It is painted on to the warts surface at weekly intervals. Larger warts need electrodessication and currettage or surgical excision.

In some cases, the warts may disappear spontaneously or by psychotherapy.

HERPEX SIMPLEX

Herpes simplex is one of the commonest viral infection caused by herpes hominis group of virus. These are of two types: (1) herpes hominish type-I-usully associated with nongenitial infection, and (2) herpes hominis type II-associated with genital infection.

The different clinical types of herpes simplex infection may be divided into two broad group:

1. *Primary herpetic infection*
   Herpetic gingivostomatitis
   Herpetic vulvovaginitiis
   Herpetic keratoconjunctivitis
   Inoculation herpes simplex
   Kaposi's varicelliform eruption (eczema herpeticum)
2. *Recurrent herpes infection*
   Recurrent herpes simplex
   Recurrent herpes progenitalis
   Recurrent herpes keratoconjunctivitis
   Recurrent herpes eczema herpeticum.

Primary Herpetic Gingivoistomatitis and Vulvovaginitis

This infection is characterized by sudden onset of round or oval superficial erosions with a well demarcated inflammatory margin present in oral cavity. Gums are red, swollen and painful. It is usually associated with fever, malaise and restlessness. Regional lymph nodes are enlarged and tender. This infection usually occurs in the first five years of life. Primary herpetic vulvovaginitis is very similar to primary herpetic gingivostomatitis.

Inoculation Herpes Simplex

It is due to direct implantation of the virus into the damaged skin, producing a painful vesiculo-pustular lesion often associated with fever and regional lymphadenopathy.

Kaposi's Varicelliform Eruption (Eczema Herpeticum)

This manifests as a sudden eruption of umblicated vesicular lesions, mainly on the face, neck, chest and upper extremities after inoculation of herpes simplex virus into a primarily diseased skin, usually atopic dermatitis. Occasionally, disease may be fatal especially in infants.

Recurrent Herpes Simplex

The latent dormant herpes virus after the primary infection can be reactivated by certain stimuli like fever, mechanical or psychological trauma, sunshine, allergy, menstruation etc., to produce recurrent manifestations. Recurrent herpes simplex infection can occur anywhere but preferred sites are the lips and the perioral areas (Herpes labialis). Clinically, it is characterized by eruption of grouped vesicular lesions on an erythematous base, usually preceded by mild pain or burning sensation. In a few days, crust is formed and complete healing takes place within 10-14 days.

Recurrent Herpes Progenitalis

It is caused by Herpes hominis virus type 2 transmitted by sexual contact. It is characterized by grouped vesicular lesions which soon get rupture to form asymptomatic or painful ulcers. Common sites are glans penis, prepuce, vulva and cervix. Recurrent infection of cervix may cause carcinoma of cervix.

Recurrent herpetic infection of eyes may lead on to keratoconjunctivitis and dendritic corneal ulcers. Eczema herpeticum may also occur as a recurrent lesion.

Treatment

Many herpetic lesions are transient and localized and need no treatment. Topical antibiotic ointments are usually prescribed to prevent secondary infections. Local application of ether, idoxuridine (5-20%), tromantidine hydrochloride (1%) and acyclovir ointment may be useful in recurrent infection. Systemic amantidine hydrochloride and acyclovir are also useful in the early stage of infection. Other modes of treatment recommended to prevent the recurrences are photoinactivation of virus using neutral red dye and by enhancing the immune mechanism giving levamisole orally.

HERPES ZOSTER

Herpes zoster is a neurodermic disease caused by varicella-zoster virus. It is the response of a partially immune host to a reactivation of the varicella virus present in the sensory neurons in latent form.

Clinical Features

Prodromal symptoms such as fever, malaise, and unilateral pain may precede the skin lesions. Skin lesions are unilateral, closely grouped, vesicular or vesiculo-pustular on an erythematous base, confining to one or more dermatomes. The lesions occur in successive crops over 5-7 days. The vesicle dries to form a crust which slowly heals without scarring in about two weeks. Regional lymph nodes are enlarged and tender. The thoracic segment is more commonly involved than other segments. Generalization is frequently in a state of immuno-suppression.

Complications

These include bacterial infections, haemorrhagic and necrotic changes, postherapetic neuralgia (seen in elderly), hemiplegia in zoster cervicalis, occular complications (conjunctivitis, keratitis, iritis) in zoster ophthalmicus and facial palsy (Ramsey Hunt Syndrome) in zoster of otic ganglion.

Treatment

For uncomplicated cases, a symptomatic treatment is required in the form of application of soothing agent like calamine lotion. Topical antibacterial agent is usually prescribed to prevent secondary infection and subsequent scarring. Systemic antibiotics may be required in certain cases. If pain is severe, analgesics may be necessary.

The risk of development of most herpetic neuralgia in elderly patients can be reduced by giving 20-30 mg of corticosteroids in the early stages.

Various modes of treatment of post-herpetic neuralgia which are worth trying include oral analgesics and antiinflammatory agents, oral carbamazepine, local anaesthetic injections, ganglion blocking agents and surgical nerve root division.

MOLLUSCUM CONTAGIOSUM

This infection is caused by a pox group of virus. It is characterized [illegible] multiple dome shaped, waxy or pearly papules with central umblication. Central core of the lesion can be easily squeezed out revealing a soft cheesy material. Children are more commonly affected. The common sites of involvement are the face, the neck, the

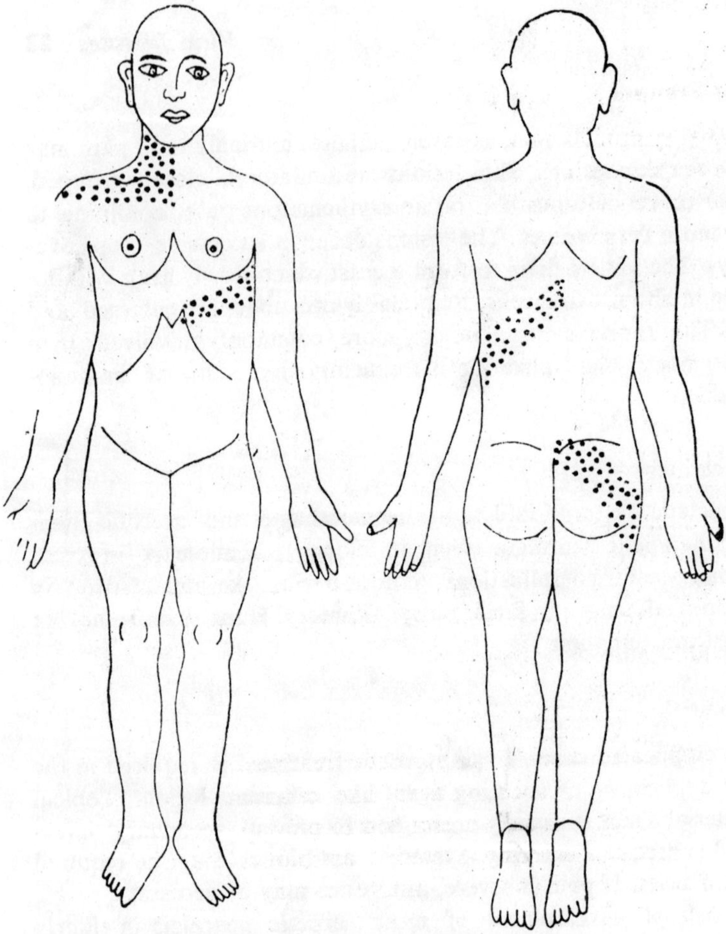

Fig. 5 Herpes Zoster: Distribution of lesions

eyelids, the genitals and the axaillae. The best treatment is to squeeze out the content and to apply phenol or trichloroacetic acid (50-100%).

5

Fungus Diseases

A fungus is a saprophytic or parasitic plant and is incapable of photosynthesizing its own organic food requirements due to lack of chlorophyll.

Despite the large number of fungi in the world, relatively few species of fungi are human pathogens. The fungi responsible for human disease may be either multicellular forming filaments known as hyphae or unicellular yeast which reproduce by budding. The fungal infections can be simply classified as follows:

1. Superficial mycoses, which affects skin and mucous membrane:

—Dermatophyte infections (Tinea)

—Candidiasis

—Pityriasis versicolor

2. Deep mycoses, which invade the living tissue and causes systemic disease:

—Madura foot

—Sporotrichosis

—Chromomycosis

SUPERFICIAL MYCOSES

Dermatophyte Infections (Tinea)

These infections are caused by multicellular filamentous fungi, the dermatophytes, which invade the dead keratinized tissues i.e. the stratum corneum of skin, hair and nail. The dermatophytes are classified into three generas-microsporum, trichophyton and epidermophyton. Microsporum species (M. audouinii) produce disease in skin and hair, trichophyton (T. violaceum, T. mentagrophyte, T. verrucosum, T. schoenleinii) in skin, hair and nail and epidermophyton (E. floccosum) in skin and nail.

Some of these dermatophytes live only on the humans (Anthropophilic), others primarily affect animals (Zoophilic) and a few dermatophytes thrive in the soil (Geophilic). Thus, dermatophyte infections may be transmitted to man from infected animal, man or soil. Poor nutrition and hygiene, a hot and humid climate, deblitating diseases, corticosteroid therapy and contact with infected animals, persons or fomites, all predispose to infection.

Dermatophyte infections are classified according to the anatomical sites of involvement. These clinical types and sites of infections are as follows:

1. Tinea capitis (Scalp)
2. Tinea barbae (Beard)
3. Tinea corporis (Body)
4. Tinea cruris (Groin)
5. Tinea manuum (Hand)
6. Tinea pedis (Foot)
7. Tinea unguium (Nail)

Tinea Capitis

Tinea capitis is the fungal infection of the scalp caused by microsporum or trichophyton species. The disease mainly affects children and is usually contracted from infected combs or hair brushes. It is manifest in following types:

1. Grey patch type: This consist of single or multiple scaly, rough, grey patches from which most of the hair have fallen leaving a few broken stumps of lusterless hair. This type is commonly produced by T. violaceum, T. tonsurans and M. audouinii.

2. Black dot type: This is caused by T. violaceum. The affected hair break off at the scalp surface giving a 'black dot' appearance to the lesions.

3. Kerion: This is a painful inflammatory boggy swelling covering small or large area of the scalp in which hair are loose and fallout or can be easily epilated. This type of reaction is commonly caused by zoophilic dermatophytes like T. mentagrophytes and T. verrucosum. Follicular scarring and partial alopecia is common after severe kerion.

4. Favus: This is characterized by multiple, concave, yellowish crusts on fungal scalp, called 'scutula'. Each crust is composed of

fungal filaments and epithelial debris and is pierced by a hair in the centre. This disease usually runs a chronic course and results in extensive cicatracial alopecia. It is commonly caused by T. schoenleinii.

Tinea Barbae

It occurs over the beard area of the face and neck. T. mentagrophyte, T. verrucosum and T. violaceum are commonly responsible. Lesions may be of kerion type as seen in T. capitis, or superficial type in which there are dry, rounded, red, scaly patches with short or brittle hairs.

Tinea Corporis

T. corporis is an infection of glaborous or nonhairy skin of the body, caused by species of Microsporum and Trichophyton. It is more commonly seen as itchy, red, circular scaly patches which clear centrally and slowly spread peripherally. The active border may show scales, populovesicles or pustules. Lesions may be single or multiple, discrete or coalesce to form polycyclic shapes.

Tinea Cruris

T. cruris is a fungal infection of the groin, thigh, perineum and perianal area. E. floccosum, T. rubrum and T. mentagrophyte are the commonest causative agents. The lesions are usually bilaterally symmetrical, itchy, well defined, erythematous, scaly patches with active borders. The active borders, may be vesicular, pustular or scaly. Central clearance is often incomplete. Satellite lesions may be present.

Tinea Manuum

Tinea manuum is a fungal infection of hand commonly caused by T. rubrum. Clinically, it is characterized by diffuse, fine scaling and hyperkeratoses of the palm. Circumscribed vesicular patches or discrete red papular and follicular scaly patches may occur, especially on the dorsal aspect. Involvement is unilateral in most of the cases.

Tinea Pedis

T. pedis is a fungal infection of the dorsum of foot, sole and interdigital spaces. T. mentagrophyte, T. rubrum and E. floccosum are the usual causative fungi. It is more commonly seen in adult males, particularly those who wear socks and shoes constantly. The infection is also transmitted via infected bathroom floors and swimming baths. There are three main clinical variants:

1. Interterigo type, characterized by scaly soddened whitish skin particularly in the space between 4th and 5th toes.

2. Vesicular type, characterized by vesicular eruptions over instep portion of the sole, toes or dorsum of the foot. The vesicles may become pustules. The lesions rupture and then dry leaving irregular collarette of scales. It is often associated with 'id' eruption of hands. T. metagrophyte is the most common fungus isolated from such lesions.

3. Squamous hyperkeratotic type, characterized by scaly hyperkeratotic lesions on the sole and sides of the foot which may be patchy or diffuse. T. rubrum is common causative agent.

Tinea Unguium

T. unguium is a fungal infection of nails usually caused by T. rubrum. Toe nails are much more frequently involved than finger nails. The infection is ordinarily limited to one or more but rarely all of the nails. It involves the soft keratin of the nail bed and later extend upward into the hard keratin of the nail plate. The infection usually begins at the lateral or distal edges of the nail causing the nail to be discoloured, thickened and distorted. The distal portion of the nail plate separates from the nail bed due to accumulation of soft keratin debris underneath.

Diagnosis of Tinea Infections

1. KOH preparation: Skin scrappings from the active edge of the lesions, nail clippings with subungual debris, or plucked hair are placed in a drop of 10-20% KOH solution on a microscopic slide, covered with a coverslip and heated gently to clear the keratin and then examined under microscope for presence of spores and hyphae.

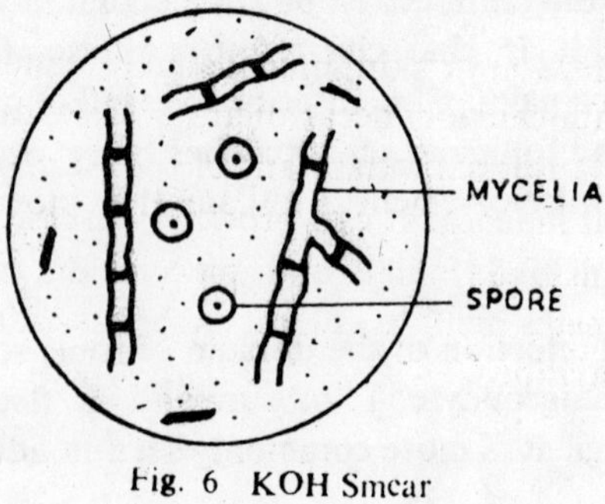

Fig. 6 KOH Smear

2. Culture: The infected material (scales, hair, nail-clippings) may be cultured on sabouraud's-dextrose-agar media for identification of species.

3. Wood's lamp: Infected hair are examined under wood's light for any fluorescence. The fungi which give fluorescence are M. canis, M. audouinii and T. schoenleinii.

Treatment of Tinea Infections

All tinea infections should be treated with topical antifungal agents and only supplemented by systemic therapy when the dermatophyte has invaded scalp, hairs or a large area of skin. Various topical antifungal agents like whitfield's ointment, Castellani's paint, clotrimazole, miconazole, econazole, tolnaftate, undecylinic acid and ciclopirox olamine have been used for treatment of dermatophyte infections. Topical agent is to be applied twice daily usually for about a month and to be continued for at least 7-10 days after the lesions have disappeared completely.

Griseofulvin and Ketoconazole are the two drugs available for sytemic therapy. Griseofulvin is given orally in the dosage of 250 mg twice a day after meals. Duration of treatment depends upon the clinical types of dermatophyte infection. T. capitis and T. pedis usually require 4 to 8 weeks therapy while T. unguium requires treatment for 4 to 8 months. Treatment of toe nail is often unsatisfactory.

Ketoconazole is a new broad-spectrum antifungal agent which is usually recommended in cases of Griseofulvin resistance and is given in a dose of 200-400 mg/day with food.

General measures include personal cleanliness, thorough drying after washing, use of clean linens and avoidance of tight fitting shoes and undergarments.

Candidiasis

Candidiasis is an infection of skin, mucous membrane and visceras, caused by candida albicans or occasionally other candida species. Candida albicans is a normal inhabitant of oral cavity, gastrointestinal tract and vaginal mucosa. It can produce disease under certain favourable conditions like trauma and maceration, antibiotics and steroid therapy, diabetes mellitus, blood dyscrasias, pregnancy, malignancies and malnutrition.

Clinical Features

Mucosal candidiasis (Thrush) produces soft white plaques on the tongue and buccal surfaces which can be scrapped off to leave a bright red moist base. Similar lesions may occur on the mucosa of the vagina (Vulvo-vaginitis) and usually associated with creamy discharge and marked local pruritis. Infection of the angle of the mouth may cause fissures (angular stomatitis). In male, glans penis and prepuce may show erythema and maceration (Balanoposthitis) through sexual contact with infected females.

Cutaneous candidiasis is characterized by moist, red macerated areas with poorly defined margins and satellite vesico-pustules. Pruritis is usually present and at times may be intense. It typically involves the body folds (Intertrigo), the napkin area in infants (Napkin dermatitis) or the nail folds (Chronic paronychia).

Diagnosis

Demonstration of candida, especially in mycelia form in KOH preparation confirms the diagnosis. Culture can be done on Sabouraud's-dextrose-agar media.

Treatment

Various topical agents such as gentian violet 1%, natamycin, haymycin, nystatin, miconazole and clotrimazole are highly effective in the treatment of candidal infection. For oral candidiasis, nystatin suspension is kept in the mouth for few minutes and then swallowed. In vulvo-vaginitis, nystatin, clotrimazole or miconazole pessaries are inserted twice daily for 2 weeks and it is advisable to give oral nystatin to prevent the recurrences.

In every patient, underlying predisposing factors should be corrected as far as possible.

Pityriasis Versicolor

Pityriasis versicolor is a mild, chronic, asymptomatic infection of the most superficial layers of the skin caused by Pityrosporum orbiculare. It is very common in warm and humid climate and usually affect young adults. It is characterized by fine, scaly, hyper or hypopigmented macules of varying sizes and shapes which appear on trunk, upper arms, shoulders and neck. Macules may become confluent to form polycyclic patches.

Diagnosis

The microscopic examination of skin scrapping in a KOH preparation reveals short hyphae and cluster of round and budding yeast cells. Scaly lesions usually show golden yellow fluorescence when examined under wood's light.

Treatment

Selenium sulphide shampoo (2.5%) is applied to the affected part at bed time and washed off next morning. Such treatment is being repeated after 5-7 days. Miconazole or clotrimazole are also effective and applied twice daily for 10-14 days. Oral ketoconazole (200-400 mg/day) may be used in cases with extensive and long standing eruptions.

2. DEEP MYCOSES

Madura Foot (Mycetoma)

Mycetoma is a chronic granulomatous condition which affects skin, subcutaneous tissue and bones. It may be Eumycetoma, caused by variety of fungi (Madurella mycetoma and Madurella grisea) or Actinomycetoma, caused by aerobic actinomycetes (Nocardia and Actinomedura medurae). The disease is common in adult males and usually occurs after trauma. The commonest site is the foot or hand but other sites may be involved.

Clinically, it is characterized by presence of firm to hard subcutaneous nodules and swellings. These nodules break open and discharge pus containing grains. There may be involvement of underlying bones and joints by the invasion of the fungus.

Diagnosis

It is made by microscopic examination of the grains from the lesion and culture of the fungi.

Treatment

Treatment of eumycetoma is usually unsatisfactory but amphotericin B and griseofulvin may be tried. In actinomycetoma, combination of dapsone with streptomycin or cotrimoxazole plus streptomycin has been reported to give good results.

In some cases, medical therapy may have to be supplemented by surgical excision, drainage and curettage of sinuses.

Sporotrichosis

It is a chronic infection of skin, subcutaneous tissue and lymph nodes, caused by Sporothrix schenckii. The lesions are usually initiated by trauma inoculating organism into subcutaneous tissue and are found mainly in farmers.

Clinically, it is characterized by presence of nodulo-ulcerative lesions in a linear fashion along the lymphatics. Regional lymphnodes may be enlarged. Rarely, sporotrichosis may disseminate via the blood stream. The diagnosis is made by histology and culture of biopsy material.

Treatment

The condition respond to oral saturated potassium iodide solution, starting with 5 to 10 drops and gradually increased to 15 drops, three times a day. When Iodides are not tolerated or are ineffective, amphotericin B is the treatment of choice. Intravenous miconazole and oral ketaconazole have also been used with some successs.

Chromomycosis

It is a cutaneous and subcutaneous mycosis caused by species of phialophora and cladosporium. Adult male agriculture workers are most often affected. The organism enters the skin after trauma.

Clinically, it is characterized by the development of multiple, indurated papulo-nodules on the foot or leg which slowly increase and take verrucous cauliflower like appearance. These lesions may ulcerate and later become secondarily infected. New crops of satellite lesions are usually seen along the path of lymphatic drainage.

Diagnosis

It is confirmed by culture or demonstration of clusters of brownish spores in biopsy material or in KOH preparation.

Treatment

Surgical excision or cryotherapy is the treatment of choice for small lesions. Systemic ketoconazole, amphotericin B or 5-fluorouracil may also be effective.

6

Eczema and Dermatitis

The term eczema and dermatitis are used synonymously to describe distinctive pattern of inflammatory response of the skin to a wide range of external and internal factors, acting singly or in combination.

The clinical presentation of eczema is variable but fairly distinctive. The major symptom of ezcema is pruritus which may be very severe. Eczema is either acute, chronic or mixed.

The cardinal signs of acute eczema are erythema, oedema, papules, vesicles, oozing, crusting and scaling. Histopathologically, the epidermis shows parakeratosis, intercellular oedema (spongiosis), vesicle formation and exocytosis. The dermis shows vascular dilatation, oedema and perivascular infilterate.

In chronic eczema lichenification hyperpigmentation and/or hypopigmentation are the prominent features. Histological changes are hyperkeratosis, parakeratosis, acanthosis, elongation of reteridges and chronic lymphocytic infiltrate in the upper dermis.

There are two major groups of eczema, exogenous and endogenous.

EXOGENOUS ECZEMAS

There are three types of exogenous eczemas: irritant dermatitis, allergic contact dermatitis and infective dermatitis (infectious eczematoid dermatitis).

Irritant Dermatitis

Irritant dermatitis is an non-immunological phenomenon resulting from contact of the skin with an irritant which chemically damages the skin. An irritant will thus cause dermatitis in most people if it is applied in sufficient concentration for a sufficient time. There are two types of irritants, strong irritants and weak irritants. Strong irritants such as acids, alkalies, caustics and strong antiseptics usually cause an acute irritant dermatitis following single exposure. Clinically, it is characterized by erythema, oedema, papules or vesicles and bullae. There may be necrosis and ulceration. Weak irritants such as detergents, soaps and cutting oils, may produce dermatitis by repeated or prolonged contact with the skin. It causes dryness, cracking and later lichenification of the skin. It occurs commonly in housewives where hands are frequently exposed to such substances.

Most irritant eczemas are confined to the area of contact. Person with dry skin, ichthyosis or atopic dermatitis are more prone to develop irritant dermatitis.

Allergic Contact Dermatitis

Allergic contact dermatitis is caused by contact of the skin with a substance to which the patient has become specifically sensitized. The substance is a simple chemical which acts as a hapten and becomes complete antigen when it combines with epidermal protein. These simple chemicals include metals such as nickel and chromium; dyes in cosmetics and clothings; rubber; plastics and resins; juices from the plants, vegetables and fruits; and medicaments. The clinical picture may be acute, chronic or mixed type. The severity of the dermatitis depends upon the dose of the antigen and the degree of the contact hypersenstitivity in the patient. There is usually a latent period of at least 1-3 days between exposure to the antigen and the development of the sensitivity. The distribution of the dermatitis corresponds to the sites of exposure to the allergens e.g. dermatitis of ear lobule from earings, dermatitis of the pressure area of soles from shoes. Predisposing factors are genetic, sensitization potential of substance, damaged skin, hyperhidrosis, humid climate and occluded areas, while malignancies, leprosy, and other deblitating diseases interfere with the development of contact dermatitis.

Infective Dermatitis (Infectious Eczematoid Dermatitis)

Infective dermatitis results from a localized sensitization to the exudate from an boil, abscess, draining ear or nose, infected wound or any secondarily infected process. It manifests as circumscribed moist, crusted and erythematous plaque studded with vesicles and pustules. The lesion is usually in direct contiguity with the primary exudative lesion. Autoinocculation is commonly seen in this condition.

ENDOGENOUS ECZEMAS

Different types of endogenous eczemas are atopic dermatitis, seborrheoic dermatitis, pompholyx, nummular or discoid eczema, pityriasis alba and lichen simplex chronicus.

Atopic Dermatitis (AD)

AD is a genetically determined disease which is frequently associated with asthma, rhinitis and hay fever in the same patient or the family. Individuals with atopic dermatitis have an increased tendency to produce reagenic (IgE) antibodies.

Atopic dermatitis usually begins in the 3rd or 4th month of life and it may continue or recur in adult life. It manifest as erythematous, papulovesicular, exudative and crusted iesions, distributed symmeterically, on the cheeks, forehead, extensors of the extremities and trunk (infantile phase). The lesion is always extremely irritable and rubbing produces a more widespread eruption. As the child grows, the distribution pattern of atopic dermatitis changes. The antecubital and popliteal fossae are invariably involved and the lesions are intensly pruritic, erythematous papules and plaques. Frictional areas such as the wrists, ankles and neck are also commonly affected. The repeated scratching gives rise to lichenification particularly on the flexures (Childhood phase). Atopic dermatitis in adults ordinarily has the same classic distribution as in children. The lesions are more lichenified and chronic (adult hood phase).

Dry skin, excessive heat, woollen clothings and emotional stress usually exacerbate atopic dermatitis. Individuals with atopic dermatitis are liable to develop anaphylactic reactions to drugs and insect bites, food allergy, and bacterial and viral infections. The course of the disease is unpredictable but spotaneous remission and relapses ar common. The majority of the patients are cleared by 10-12 years.

Seborrhoeic Dermatitis

It is a chronic recurrent, inflammatory dermatosis of unknown aetiology. It is associated frequently with oily or greasy skin with patulous

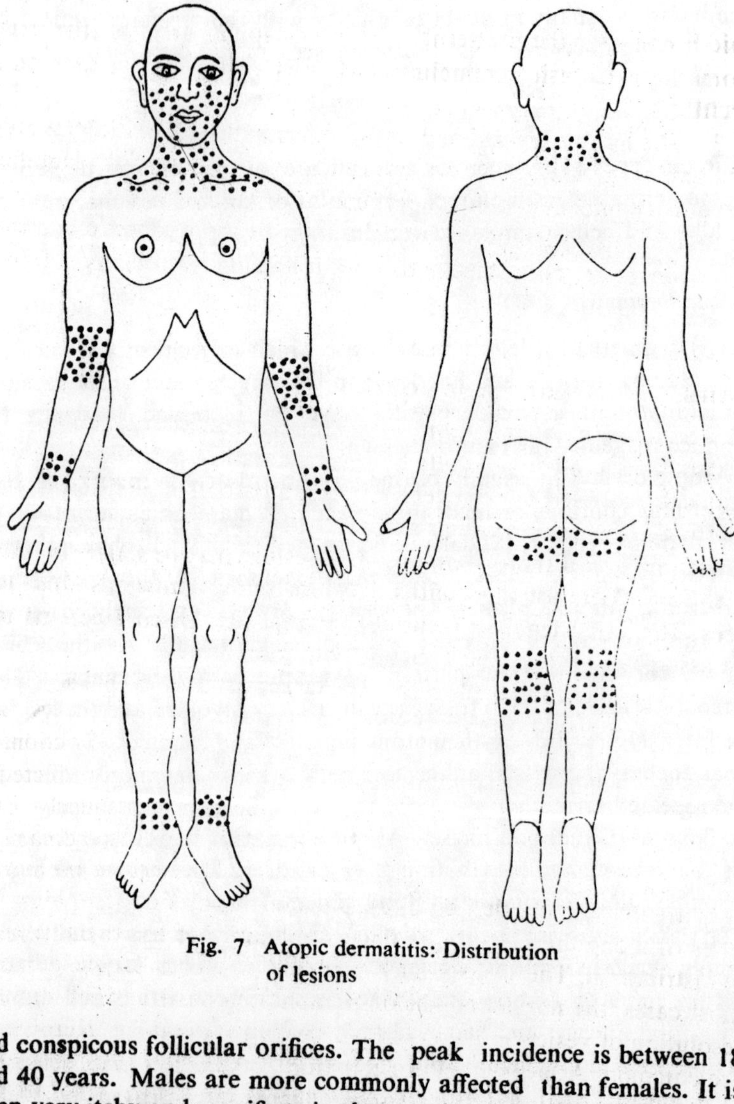

Fig. 7 Atopic dermatitis: Distribution of lesions

and conspicous follicular orifices. The peak incidence is between 18 and 40 years. Males are more commonly affected than females. It is often very itchy and manifests in three main patterns of dermatitis which may occur in any combination.

1. There is varying degree of diffuse or patchy redness and greasy scaling on the scalp, forehead, eyebrows, eyelashes, nasolabial folds, retroauricular areas and beard area.

2. There are small erythematous, follicular papules covered with greasy scales which enlarge and coalesce to form a characterstic reta-

loid lesion over the presternal and interscapular area of the trunk. Sometimes, a rash resembling pityriasis rosea may be seen on the trunk.

3. The lesions are red and moist, often with maceration involving the axillae, groins, natal cleft, submammary areas and umbilicus. Secondary infection with candida albicans is very common.

Individuals with seborrhoeic dermatitis are more prone to pyococcal infections like boil, blephritis and folliculitis, especially of beard region.

Nummular Eczema (Discoid Eczema)

It is a common inflammatory dermatoses of unknown aetiology. It occurs chiefly in young adults but may be seen in patients of all ages. It is characterized by well defined, round patches of erytherma studded with vesicles or erosions and crusting, occuring commonly on the dorsal surface of the extremities. The lesions may be single or multiple. They often last for months or years with remissions and relapses. The lesion tends to recur at the same site. Discoid eczema may be associated with atopic dermatitis.

Dry skin, emotional stress and focal sepsis usually precipitate or aggravate the condition.

Pompholyx

Pompholyx is an acute, recurrent, non inflammatory vesicular disease of the hands and feet. It usually presents in young adults. The lesions are itchy, multiple, small, deep seated vesicles on the palms and soles or along the sides of the fingers and more or less symmeterical in distribution. The vesicles may coalesce to form large bullae. In most cases, the normal course of pompholyx consists of spontaneous resolution of vesicular lesions in 2-3 weeks with scaling. Recurrences are common. Attacks are more common in summer and often precipitated by emotional stress, fungus infection of the feet or ingested allergens. Pompholyx is also called as dyshidrosis because it is often associated with hyperhidrosis.

Pityriasis Alba

Pityriasis alba is a non-specific dermatitis of unknown origin. It manifests mainly on the cheeks in young children as single or multi-

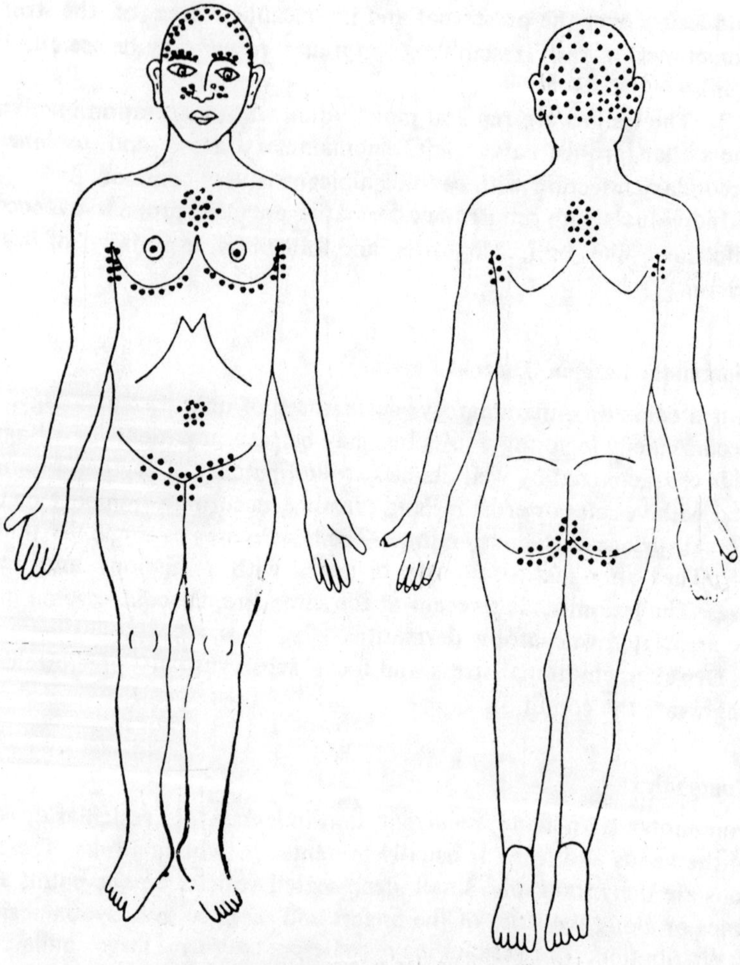

Fig. 8 Seborrhoeic dermatitis: Distribution of lesions

ple, round or oval hypopigmented macules with fine scaling. It can occur at anytime of the year, but is more common in winter.

The condition is usually self limiting.

Lichen Simplex Chronicus (LSC)

LSC is a chronic localized type of eczema characterized by the presence of one or more well defined lichenified patches. It occurs mainly in adults and females are affected more often than males. The

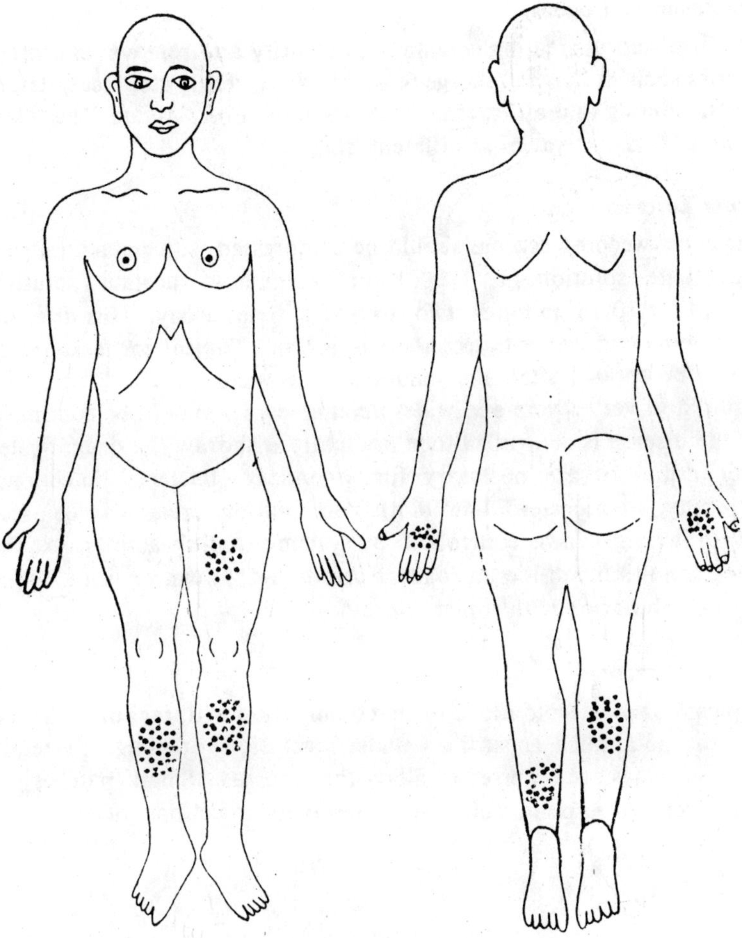

Fig. 9 Nummular eczema: Distribution of lesions

common sites are the nape of the neck, the ankles, the lower legs, the forearm, and the perineal areas.

Lichenified patches are produced as a result of continuous scratching and rubbing. The rubbing is usually initiated by psychological factors or pruritic dermatoses. These patches are extremely pruritic and continual scratching leads to more inflammation which leads to more itching, thus completing a vicious circle in which LSC may last for years.

Treatment of Eczemas

The first step in treating eczema is to identify and remove causative factors such as contact allergens, stress, focal sepsis etc. Heat, detergents, rubbing and all external irritants should be avoided. The treatment of eczemas varies at different stages.

Acute Eczemas

The acute weeping eczema should be compressed with potassium permanganate solution (1 : 10000) or aluminium acetate solution (1-5%) for 10-15 minutes two to three times a day. This dries up the eczema and prevents secondary infection. Topical corticosterioids should be applied after the compresses. Systemic steroids may be required in very severe and widespread cases. It should be continued till the disease is controlled then gradually withdraw the drug. Systemic antiboitics are necessary for secondary bacterial infections. Topically, a coticosteroid antibiotic combination cream can be used. Severe itching can be controlled by systemic antihistamines. As the acute condition subsides, a coal tar cream (1-5%) can be used alone or in combination with topical steroid.

Chronic Eczema

Topical corticosteroid alone or in combination with tar or salicylic acid can be applied as such or under occlusion dressing. Systemic antihistamines are required to allay the pruritis. Small patches of lichenification respond well to intralesional injections of corticosteroids.

7
Psoriasis

Psoriasis is a common, chronic inflammatory disease of the skin, characterized by erythematous papules and plaques surmounted by silvery white scale.

Aetiopathogenesis

The disease can involve any group but peak incidence is seen in between 15-40 years. Both sexes are equally affected. Exact aetiology is unknown, probably it is multifactorial. The genetic basis of psoriasis is based on the familial incidence of psoriasis and increased prevalence of certain HLA antigens (B13, B16 and B17). Certain provocating factors like trauma, infection, emotional upset, climate changes, drugs (chloroquine and betablockers) and hormonal variation may precipitate or exacerbate the disease.

The characteristic pathophysiological event in psoriasis is increased epidermopoiesis. The increased level of cyclic GMP and variable level of cyclic AMP have been found in psoriatic lesions. Immunological phenomenon may take part in the pathogenesis of the disease.

Pathology

Histology is characterized by

1. Parakeratosis and acanthosis
2. Elongation of rete ridges
3. Broadening of lower ends of rete ridges
4. Thinning of suprapapillary portion
5. Elongation of dermal papillae
6. Oedema and dilated capillaries in upper dermis.
7. Presence of munro-microabscesses

Clinical Features

The lesions are asymptomatic or mildly itchy, erythematous papules and plaques covered with loosely adherent silvery scales. When scratched lightly with a glass slide, the silver colour of scales becomes more prominent. Further scratching causes pin point bleeding (Auspitz's sign). The common affected sites are the elbows, the knees, the scalp and the sacrum. The lesions vary in shape and size and some lesions may merge to form annular or gyrate figures. Isomorphic lesions of psoriasis may develop at the site of trauma (Koebner phenomenon).

In some cases, the nails are also involved showing thimble pitting, yellow discolouration and onycholysis or thickening and ridging of the nail plate.

The disease is chronic with spontaneous remission and relapses at variable intervals. Attacks are more common in winter than summer.

There are many clinical variants of psoriasis:

Guttate Psoriasis

It is characterized by sudden appearance of drop size, erythematous, scaly papules over the trunk and the extremities. It is usually seen in children following a streptococcal upper respiratory infection..

Flexural Psoriasis

Psoriasis in body folds loses its characteristic scales and manifests as itchy, smooth, shiny erythematous lesio

Pustular Psoriasis

There are two clinical types: (1) palmoplantar pustular psoriasis is characterized by presence of erythematous and scaly plaques studded with sterile pustules on palms or soles; (2) generalized pustular psoriasis (Von Zumbusch type) is characterized by an acute eruption of a generalized pustular rash in a psoriatic patient, usually associated with marked constitutional symptoms. It may be precipitated by infections, withdrawal of systemic corticosteriods or irritant applications.

Psoriatic Arthropathy

It is chronic inflammatory arthritis in patients with psoriasis, which chiefly involves the distal interphalangeal joints. It is usually associated with severe psoriasis and nail changes. Sometime, there is extensive mutilation of the joints of extremities.

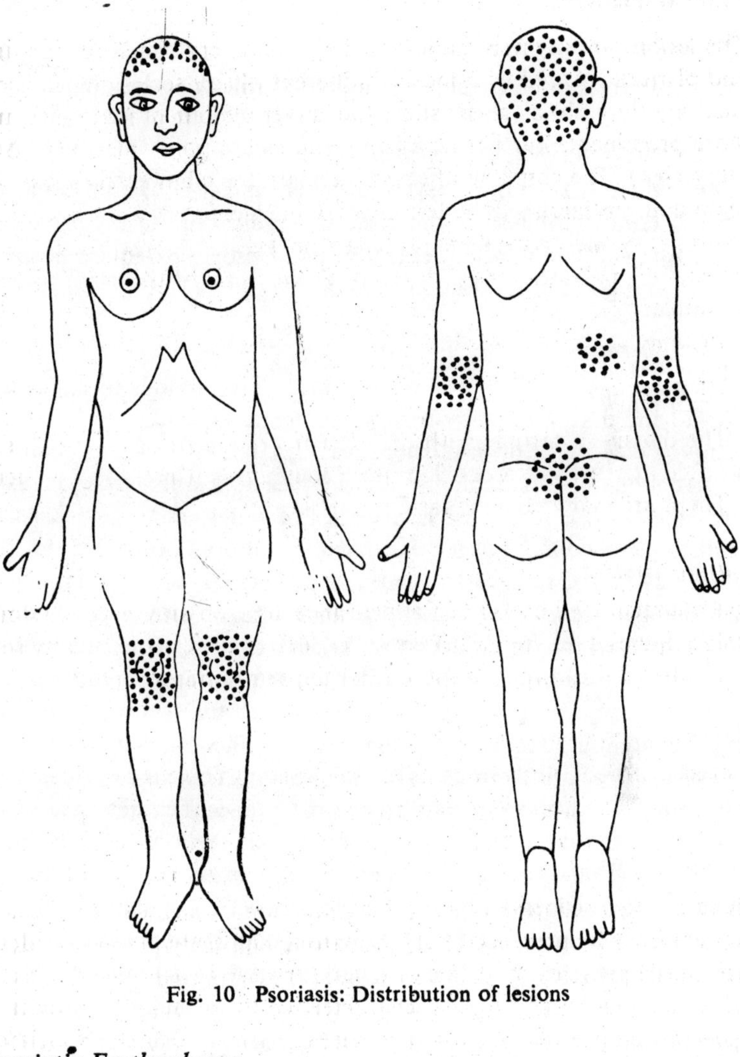

Fig. 10 Psoriasis: Distribution of lesions

Psoriatic Erythroderma

It is characterized by generalized erythema and scaling of the body surface, may occur spontaneously or as a reaction to topical therapy. Some typical lesions of psoriasis can always be detected in this variety.

Seborrhoeic dermatitis, lichen simplex chronicus, lichen planus, diabetes mellitus, gout, malabsorption syndrome and hypocalcemia may be seen in association with psoriasis.

Treatment

The treatment can be considered under the following headings:

General and Non-Specific Measures

These include reassurance, psychotherapy and use of mild tranquillizers to remove the fear of the disease. Eradication of the provocating factors is often helpful. Severe forms of psoriasis require hospitalization and good general nursing care.

Topical Therapy

The topical agents which are most useful, are various forms of tar, salicylic and diathranol, emollients and corticosteroids.

Liquor picis carb. or crude coal tar (5-10%) in various bases is effective alone or in combination with other adjuvants, such as salicylic acid (3-5%). Coal tar is the basis of widely used Goeckerman regimen which consists of local application of crude coal tar to the skin for 24 hours, then after a bath, a ultraviolet therapy is given. This regimen clears widespread psoriasis within 3-4 weeks. Dithranol can be used in concentration of 0.05%, to 0.5% as an alternative to tar. In the standard Ingram technique, the patient is exposed to ultraviolet rays after a tar bath and the lesions are then painted with a paste containing 0.05 to 0·1% diathranol. This regimen also clears most of the psoriatic lesions within 3 weeks. Topical corticosteroid application is indicated in psoriasis of scalp, face, flexures and genitalias. Recalcitrant patches require occlusive therapy with corticosteroids. Sometimes patches are anatomically unsuitable for occlusion and these may be treated by intralesional injection of steroid.

In acute and unstable forms of psoriasis, bland preparations such as calamine lotion with or without oil, liquid paraffin should be applied.

Systemic Therapy

Systemic medications include methotrexate, corticosteroids and psoralens. Methotrexate is indicated in psoriatic erythroderma, psoriatic arthropathy, generalized pustular psoriasis and intractable and crippling psoriasis. It is given in dosage of 0.2 to 0.4 mg/kg body weight either as a single weekly dose or it can be divided into 3 parts given 12 hourly over 36 hours period. Hepatic, renal and bone marrow functions of the patient should be assessed at a regular intervals. Corticosteroids have no place in the management of psoriasis except in severe form of the disease where administration of methotrexate is contraindicated. Another mode of systemic therapy is by oral psoralen and ultraviolet radiation A (PUVA). 8-methoxypsoralen is given orally in a dose of 0.6 mg/kg body weight, followed 2 hours later by exposure to ultraviolet A light.

Other systemic drugs like etretinate, razoxane, hydroxyures and azathioprine are also useful in the treatment of psoriasis.

8

Lichen Planus, Pityriasis Rosea and Exfoliative Dermatitis

LICHEN PLANUS

Definition

Lichen planus is a subacute or a chronic dermatosis with obscure aetiology and characteristic cutaneous and sometimes mucosal lesions.

Aetiology

Exact aetiology is not known. Different theories like autoimmune, infective, genetic and psychosomatic have been incriminated. Recently the presence of lymphocytic infiltration (T cells) in the dermis suggest an immunological involvement. Increased frequency of HLA-B 7 and HLA A3 have also been seen in cases of lichen planus.

Pathology

Important pathological changes are: Hyperkeratosis, focal hypergranulosis, irregular acanthosis, liquefaction degeneration of basal layer, flattening of rete ridges in the centre with increased length at the edges giving a saw tooth appearance and dense band like infiltrate of lymphocytes in the dermis hugging the epidermis.

Clinical Features

Onset is insidious in most of the cases. It is charecterized by pruritic, purple, polygonal, plain top, papular lesions (5 Ps). The surface of the papule is marked by white dots or lines (whickham's striae). Mild scaling may be present. Appearance of isomorphic lesions may be seen at the site of trauma or a scratch (Koebner phenomenon). Annular lesions which are formed either by group of papules or by a single papule showing clearance in thc centre, may be encountered.

The lesions are usually distributed bilateral and symmeterical over symmetrical flexural aspect of forearm and wrist, legs, waist, penis and oral mucous membrane.

On the legs, the lesions are larger with hyperkeratotic surface and this type of lesion is sometimes referred to as hypertrophic lichen planus. Sometimes the desease is limited to the hair follicles giving rise to a follicular eruption and if there lesions are present on scalp, there may be patchy, cicatricial loss of hairs. Occasionally, lichen planus lesions may give rise to a bullae.

In most of the cases, papules flatten after a few month leaving behind hyperpigmentation which persist, for months and years.

Oral mucous membrane lesions are commonly seen in the form of white streaks forming lacy net work in 30-70% of the cases. Occasionally, ulcerative lesions may occur on the buccal mucosa. Other mucous membranes may also be involved. Nails are involved in about 10% of the cases and changes include thinning of nail plate, longitudinal ridging, pterygium formation, subungual hyperkerotosis or occasionally complete loss of nail plate.

Treatment

Treatment is mainly symptomatic. Antihistamines are given to combat itching. For milder cases topical corticosteroid is useful. In severe cases, occlusive dressing with corticosteroid and systemic corticosteroids (20-30 mg daily) may be needed. For few localized and hyperkeratotic lesion, interalesional corticosteroid is effective. The oral lesions can be treated by keeping the soluble tablets of corticosteroids in the oral cavity, 3-4 times a day.

LICHENOID DRUG ERUPTION

Lichenoid drug eruption is induced by heavy metals, PAS, streptomycin, INH, tolbutamide, chlorpropamide, methyl dopa, paraphenylene diamine etc. It is characterized by typical lichen planus like lesions with more scaling and presence of eosinophils in the infilrate.

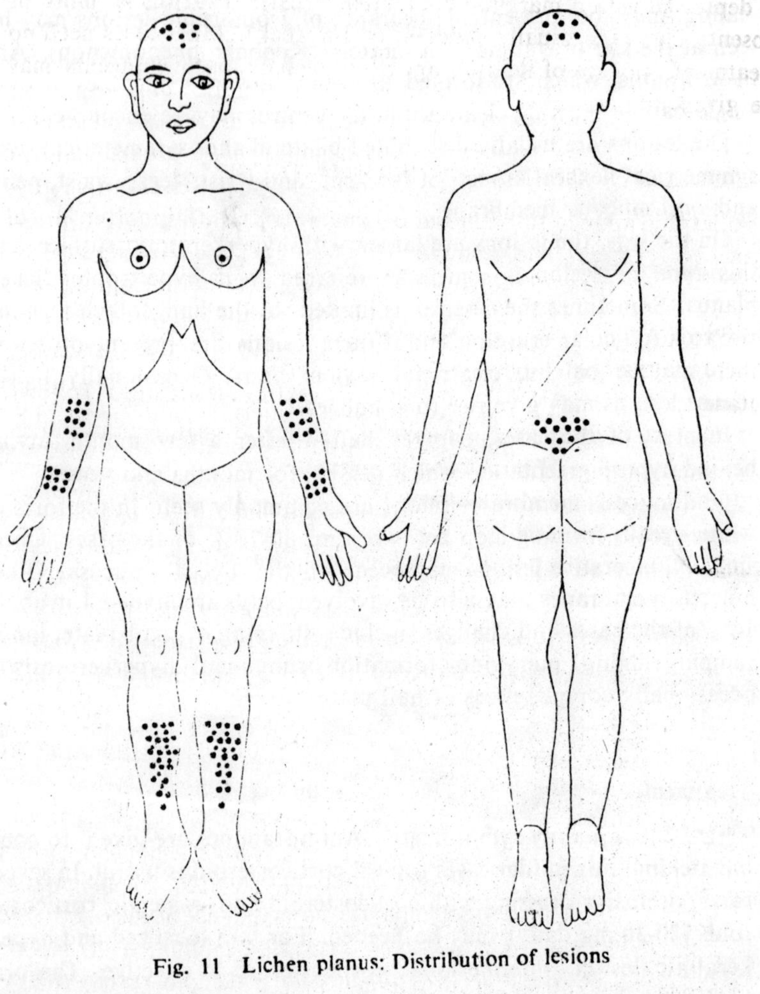

Fig. 11 Lichen planus: Distribution of lesions

PITYRIASIS ROSEA

Pityriasis rosea is a common, benign, self limiting disease of unknown aetiology, affecting children and young adults. The initial lesion is usually the 'herald patch', 2 to 6 cm in diameter, situated on the trunk, upper arms or thighs. This herald patch is followed after an interval of 5 to 15 days by a generalized eruption of small, oval, erythematous and scaly lesions, mainly on the trunk in a bilateral and symmetrical fashion. The long axis of the lesions follow the rib lines on the back to give a 'christmas-tree' appearance. Centre of the lesion is depressed with a marginal collarette of scales. Pruritus is mild or absent. The rash usually fades after 4-8 weeks. Most cases need no treatment. In case of itching, antipruritic and soothing agents may be given.

EXFOLIATIVE DERMATITS (ERYTHRODERMA)

This term is applied to universal or almost universal involvement of skin with erythema and scaling.

Aetiology

Erythroderma is always secondary or reactive process to underlying cutaneous or systemic disease. Causes of erythroderma are as follows:

1. Primary cutaneous diseases: Eczema, psoriasis, ichthyosiform dermatoses and pemphigus foliaceous.
2. Malignancies: Mycosis fungoides, Hodgkin's disease, lymphomas and leukaemias.
3. Drugs: Heavy metals, antimalarials, barbiturates and sulphonamides.
4. Idiopathic.

Clinical Features

The onset of erythroderma may be acute or gradual. The entire skin becomes erythematous, oedematous and scaly. The scales may be large or fine and bran like. The skin is thickened and feels hot. It is accompanied by fever with chills and rigors. Pruritus is generally present. Regional lymph nodes are usually enlarged. The clinical picture may be modified according to the underlying diseases. In severe and and longstanding cases, scalp and body hair may be shed and the nails develop transverse grooves.

Chronic generalized erythroderma may develop a variety of systemic problems which include interference with body temperature regulation, congestive cardiac failure, electrolyte and fluid imbalance, hypoalbuminaemia and iron deficient anaemia. Course and prognosis largely depend on nature and response of underlying process to the appropriate therapy.

Treatment

General measures include hospitalization of the patient, good nursing care, monitoring of fluid and electrolyte balance, regulation of body temperature and intake of high protein diet.

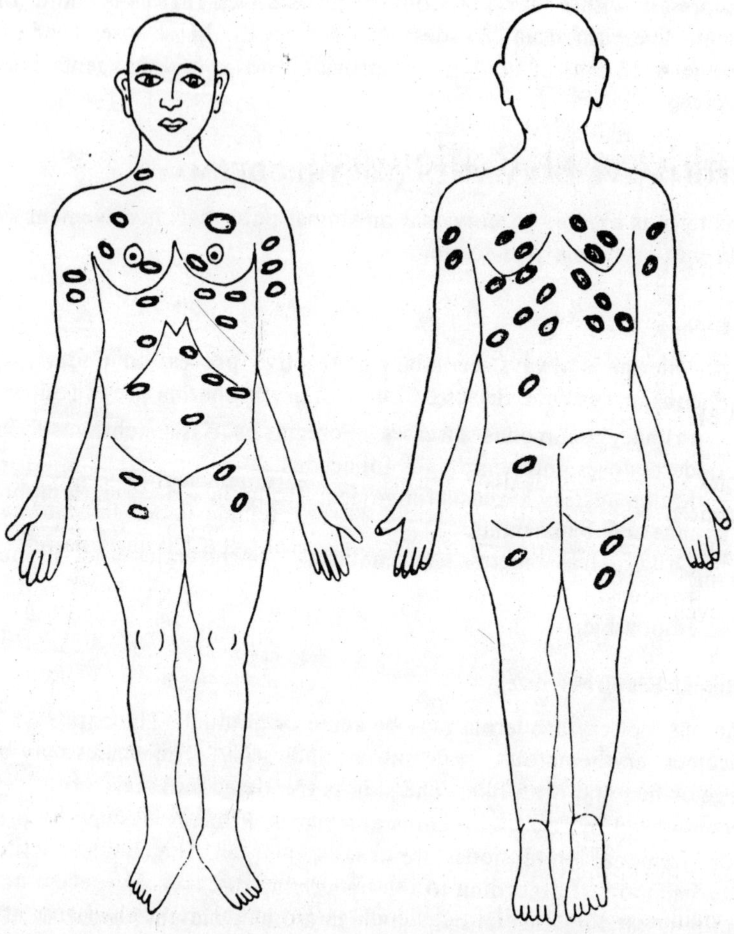

Fig. 12 Pityriasis rosea: Distribution of lesions

Systemic corticosteroids are necessary in majority of the patients. An initial dose of 40-60 mg of prednisolone per day is given to control the disease. Once the disease is controlled, the dose of prednisolone should be gradually tappered off. Topical therapy in most of the cases include daily bath with saline or oat meal powder suspension followed by application of emollients.

Systemic antibiotics are usually required to control secondary infections. Removal of cause and specific treatment of underlying cutaneous and systemic disease is required wherever necessary.

9

Scabies and Pediculosis

SCABIES

Scabies is a contagious disease caused by Sarcoptes scabei hominis, a tiny mite: male being 0.2 × 0.15 mm and female 0.4 × 0.3 mm in measurement. They are whitish hemispherical mites having 4 pairs of very short legs.

Life cycle

♂ + ♀ ⟶ Fertilized ♀ ⟶ (Burrows) Eggs ⟶ (3-4 days) Larvae ⟶ Mite

(Eggs to Mite: 14-17 days)

Male mite dies after copulation.

Clinical Features

The main complaint is itching which is worse at night. Incubation period is usually 2-3 weeks.

Skin lesions of scabies can be of three types:

(a) Lesions due to presence of mites are vesicles and burrows. Burrow is pathognomonic lesion which is 'S' shaped passage (5-15 mm), traversed by mite. It occurs most frequently on anterior aspect of wrists, the ulnar border of hand, interdigital webs, penis and palms and soles in infants. The vesicles are usually seen at the end of burrows.

(b) Lesions due to allergic sensitivity are small urticarial papules, excoriation marks and rarely inflammatory nodules, usually seen on lower abdomen, the buttocks, the thighs and the scrotum.

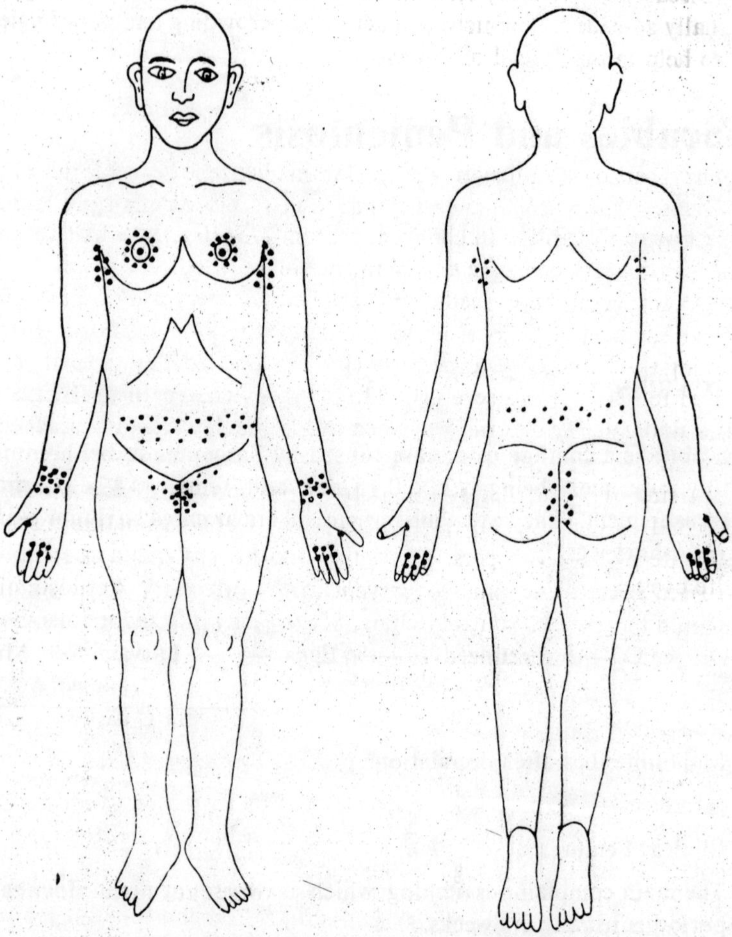

Fig. 13 Scabies: Distribution of lesions

(c) Lesions due to complication can be pustular, impetiginous and eczematous. Rarely glomerulonephritis may complicate the pyoderma.

Other members of the family may also show similar manifestation. Sites of predilection are interdigital webs, the anterior aspect of wrist joint, the ulnar side of forearm, anterior fold of axillae, elbows, lower abdomen, penis and scrotum, arround the nipples in women and palms, soles and scalp in infants.

Disease is commonly seen in children but can affect any age. It usually spreads by intimate contact. Over crowding and poor hygiene also help in the spread of disease.

Treatment

Benzyl benzoate emulsion (25%), Gamma benzene hexachloride (1%), Monosulphiran (25%) and crotomiton (10%) are commonly used in treatment of scabies. In children, crotomiton (10%) and half strength of 25% Benzyl benzoate emulsion should be used.

After a scrub bath, medicine is applied all over body below neck. Next day again the patient is asked to apply the medicine without taking the bath and changing the clothes. On 3rd day patient is advised to take again a scrub bath followed by change of clothings. All the under garments and bed linen should be laundered or washed in boiling water,

A single treatment is sufficient but a second treatment should be advised only after an interval of 7 days, if re examination discloses definite evidence of persistant infection. All the contacts should be treated at the same time to prevent cross infection. Antihistamines should be given to control itching. Secondarily infected lesions should be treated with suitable antibiotics.

Norwegian Scabies

This form of scabies usually occurs in the mentally retarded and immunosuppressed. This is characterized by asymptomatic hyperkeratotic and crusted lesions usually present over trunk, limbs, palms and soles. Such cases are highly contagious.

PEDICULOSIS

Pediculosis is an infestation caused by lice. There are three distinct types of lice according to the area infested:

1. Pediculus humanus capitis (Head Louse)
2. Pediculus humanus corporis (Body Louse)
3. Phthirus pubis (Pubic Louse).

Pediculosis Capitis

P. capitis is caused by pediculus humanus capitis which is 3-4 mm in length and light brown in colour, usually preferes the scalp but may rarely live on beard and other hairy areas. It is transmitted by close contact or through combs or brushes. Poor personal hygiene is also an important predisposing factor. It is commonly seen in school children, especially those with long hair.

The patient complains of severe itching around the back and the sides of the scalp. Secondary bacterial infection, eczematization and regional lymphadenopathy are common complications. The diagnosis can be confirmed by the demonstration of adult lice or by presence of small white nits (eggs) firmly attached to a hair shaft.

Treatment

It consists of application of 25% benzyl benzoate emulsion, 1% Gamma benzene hexachloride or 0.5% malathion on to the scalp hair. Next morning, the hair should be washed with a shampoo or soap. Nits may be removed with a special fine toothed comb. Treatment should be repeated after a week so as to kill the lice that may have hatched out of the nits. Secondary infections and eczematization should be treated before specific therapy.

Pediculosis Corporis

Pediculosis corporis is caused by Pediculus humanus corporis which is morphologically indistinguishable from head louse and it lives in the seams of the under clothes. It is commonly seen in individuals with grossly neglected poor hygiene and can be transmitted by close contact.

The patient will have severe itching with pinpoint macular or papular lesions, scratch marks, crusting and hyperpigmentation over the trunk and the shoulders.

Treatment

It consists of disinfection of clothes with 10% DDT, 1% Gammabenzene hexa-chloride or 0.5% malathion. Clothings may also be sterilized by boiling or by use of a hot iron especially over the seams.

Pediculosis Pubis

It is caused by Phthirus pubis, which usually inhabits the anogenital area, the axillae, the eyelashes and the eyebrows. Infestation is often transmitted by sexual contact or through fomites.

It causes intense itching and later secondary infection and eczematization may occur. Bluish grey macule may be seen on the thighs.

or lower abdomen. The nits are attached to the pubic hair or the hair of the regions mentioned.

Treatment

It is same as that of pediculosis capitis. Pediculosis of eyelashes can be treated by application of a one per cent ointment of yellow oxide of mercury.

10

Bullous Disorders

Bullae are circumscribed elevations of the epidermis containing clear fluid. It may arise at the dermoepidermal junction or at varying depth within the epidermis.

A primarily pathological event is the impairment or loss of intercellular coherence in the epidermis or dermoepidermal adherence which may be basically caused by genetically determined defects, immunological reactions and various infective or chemical agents. The various bullous disorders are classified as follows:

1. Congenital: Epidermolysis bullosa.
2. Immunological: Pemphigus, Pemphigoid, Dermatitis herpetiformis, Benign chronic bullous dermatosis of childhood, Herpes gestationis
3. Infective: Staphylococcal scalded skin syndrome, Impetigo, Vericella
4. Unknown aetiology: Erythema multiforme, Subcorneal pusular dermatosis, Toxic epidermal necrolysis.

PEMPHIGUS

Pemphigus is a group of chronic bullous disorders in which histologically, there is lack of cohesion between epidermal cells with subsequent separation (acantholysis) to form intraepidermal cleft and bullae. There are two major variants of pemphigus based on the level of intraepidermal cleft.

1. Pemphigus vulgaris and its variant, pemphigus vegetans due to suprabasal cleft.
2. Pemphigus foliaceous and its rare variant, pemphigus erythematosus due to subcorneal cleft.

Pemphigus Vulgaris and Pemphigus Vegetans

Pemphigus vulgaris is the most common variant of pemphigus, in which bullae apper incrops on apparently normal skin and mucous membrane.

Aetiology

It is of world wide distribution but is more common in Jews. It usually involves the age group of 20-40 years, but can affect any age group. Both sexes are equally affected. In pemphigus there is an autoimmune mechanism which is responsible for acantholysis, the basic pemphigus change. Pemphigus is sometimes associated with other autoimmune disorders. Increased prevalence of HLA-A 10 and HLA-DRW 4 have been reported in cases of pemphigus vulgaris.

Histologically, the earliest change is the loss of coherence between the epidermal cells due to dissolution of intercellular cement substance (acantholysis). This leads to the formation of clefts and bullae in a predominantly suprabasal location. The bullae cavity may contain few or multiple acantholytic cells.

Immunofluorescent studies show deposition of IgG antibiodies in the intercellular spaces of epidermis of both involved and univolved skin.

Clinical Features

The onset is insidious. The disease usually starts with painful erosions in the oral mucosa which may precede the skin lesions by several months. Skin lesions are characterized by eruption of flaccid bullae on apparently normal skin which breaks easily leaving raw, denuded areas of skin. These erosions are painful, bleed easily and show a little tendency to healing. Bullae usually come in crops. A shearing force applied to the normal appearing skin surface in adjacent areas causes skin to slip (Nikolsky's sign). Bullae formation can occur at any site but it characteristically involves the face, trunk, pressure points and interteriginous areas.

The lesions heal slowly by hyperpigmentation. Remissions and relapses are fairly common at irregular intervals. But the disease ends sooner or later in death.

Pemphigus Vegetans

It is a rare variant of pemphigus vulgaris, characterized by presence of hypertrophic, vegetative lesions, which appear to arise from denuded bullae. Common sites of involvement are the flexures and the mucocutaneous junction. It is commonly seen in patients with greater resistance to the disease. Prognosis is better than pemphigus vulgaris.

Diagnosis

1. *Tzanck Test*

A smear is obtained from the floor of a fresh intact bulla with the help of a blunt blade and is stained with Geimsa or Leishman stain. Acantholytic cells can be demonstrated in the smear. These cells are rounded with large nuclei and condensed cytoplasm. Some cells show a perinuclear halo.

2. *Skin Biopsy*

Biopsy of an early fresh intact bulla will show typical histological features.

3. IgG antibodies to the intercellular areas can be demonstrated by direct immunofluorescent technique.

Treatment

Systemic corticosteroids are given in dosage between 80-120 mg daily for a week or so to suppress the disease. Once the lesions starts healing and no new lesions appear, dose of corticosteroids can be gradually reduced to a maintenance level. Immunosuppressive agents like azathioprine, cyclophosphamide and methotrexate have also been used to lessen the dose of corticosteroids. In routine instances, corticosteroids may be stopped completely, and the patient may be controlled by immunosuppressive agents only.

The local treatment of the skin lesions consists of compresses with potassium permanganate followed by application of 1% gention violet or antibiotic cream. Application of topical corticosteroid with antibiotic may also be beneficial. Sterilized veseline gauze dressing is usually recommended for extensive raw areas. Systemic antibiotics should be given if there is infection.

For painful mouth lesions, xylocaine viscous may be applied before every meal and thus the patient can have an adequate intake of fluids and foods.

Pemphigus Foliaceous and Pemphigus Erythematosus

Pemphigus Foliaceous

It is a superficial, less severe from of pemphigus characterized by thin roofed, flaccid blisters which rupture easily leaving shallow erosions that heal with crusting and scaling. The distribution usually favours the 'seborrhoeic' sites, scalp, face and upper chest. The process may become generalized giving an appearance of exfoliative dermatitis. Mucosal involvement is unusual and the prognosis is better than in pemphigus vulgaris. This is usually seen between 30 and 50 years of age but not uncommon in children.

Histologically, acantholysis occurs high in the epidermis, in or near the granular cell layer. Immunofluorescent studies show antibodies against the intercellular substance.

Pemphigus Erythematosus

It is an uncommon variant of pemphigus foliaceous with the erythematous scaly lesions on the nose, cheeks and ears resembling lupus erythematosus. The lesions may sometimes be present in seborrhoeic dermatitis distribution. Immunofluorescent studies show deposition of intercellular antibodies in the epidermis in addition to immunoglobulin deposits at the dermoepidermal junction.

Treatment

Pemphigus foliaceous or erythematosus may be controlled by topical corticosteroid alone either with or without polythene occlusion. Systemic therapy with low dosage of corticosteroids may be required in some cases. Dapsone has also been used in treatment of pemphigus foliaceous.

PEMPHIGOID

This is an uncommon autoimmune disease occuring in elderly people.

Clinical Features

It begins with tense bullae, occasionally haemorrhagic on an erythematous or urticarial base on flexures. The bulla may remain intact for several days and if ruptures, healing is usually rapid and there is no tendency for the denuded area to spread peripherally. The mucous membranes are rarely affected. It is sometimes associated with malignancy particularly lymphomas. The course of the disease is variable with remissions and relapses. Histologically, there is subepidermal bulla, without acantholysis. Dermis shows inflammatory infiltrate, mainly consists of eosinophils and neutrophils. The immunofluorescent studies show IgG antibodies directed against the basement membrane.

Treatment

Treatment is same as for pemphigus vulgaris except that much lower dosages of corticosteroids (40-60 mg day) are required to control the disease process. Immunosuppressive agents like cyclophosphamide and azathioprine may be used in combination with corticosteroids. Dapsone may also be of value in some cases.

DERMATITIS HERPETIFORMIS (DH)

DH is an uncommon, autoimmune disease affecting skin and rarely the mucous membrane. It usually occurs in young adult males but occasionaly affects children. There is increased prevalence of HLA B8 and HLA DRW3 in patients of DH.

Clinical Features

The onset may be acute or gradual. The characteristic lesions are intensely itchy, papular, urticarial or papulovesicular on an erythematosus base which have a marked tendency for grouping. The distribution of these lesions is usually bilateral and symmetrical. Common sites are elbows, knees, buttocks, shoulders and sacral areas. The lesions frequently heal with hypo or hyperpigementation. The course of the disease is variable with remissions and relapses. DH has been found to be associated with gluten sensitivity enteropathy and thyroid disease.

Histologically, there is a subepidermal bulla with peribullous neutrophillic and eosinophilic papillary microabscesses. The immunofluoroscent studies show deposition of IgA antibodies at the tips of the dermal papillae.

Treatment

Dapsone is the drug of choice. The initial dose is 200-400 mg daily which produces dramatic clearance of the lesions and subsidence of itching within a few days. When the disease is controlled, the dose should be gradually reduced to a maintainence dose of 25-50 mg per

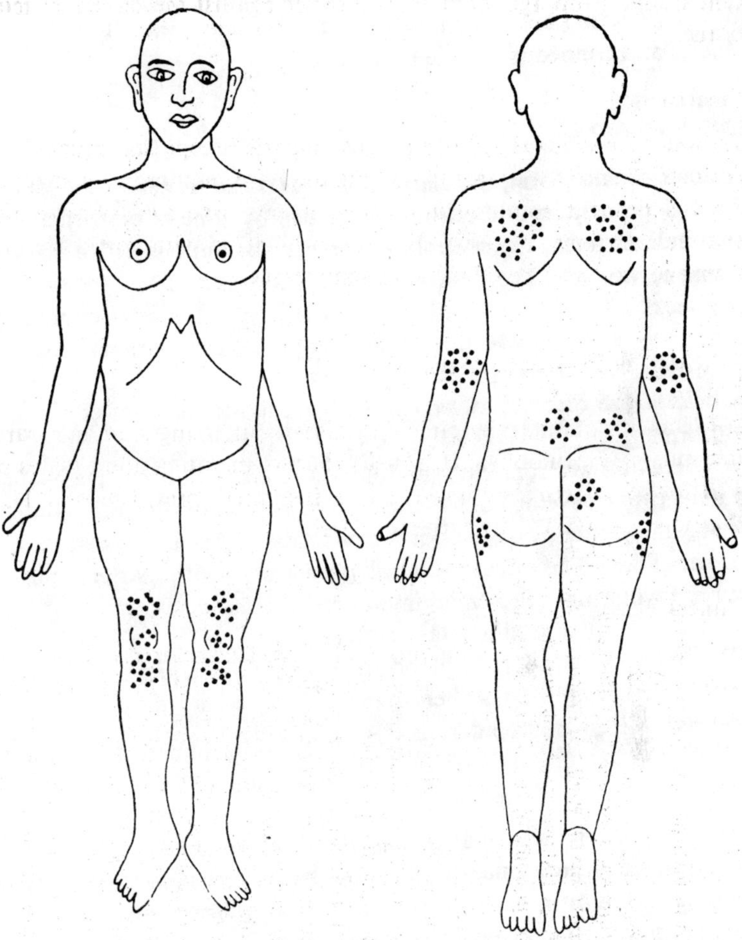

Fig. 14 Dermatitis herpetiformis: Distribution of lesions

day. Those few patients not helped by dapsone may respond well to sulphapyridine (1.5 to 2 mg/day). Gluten free diet may also be beneficial.

ERYTHEMA MULTIFORME

Erythema multiforme is a common distinctive reaction pattern of the skin and mucous membrane, secondary to variety of known or unknown factors such as infections (Herpes simplex, fungal, bacterial), drugs (long acting sulphonamide, barbiturates and penicilline), malignancies and connective tissue disorders.

Clinical Features

In maculopapular form, the classical lesions is the target lesion which has a cynotic or purpuric centre surrounded by zone of erythema. In vesico-bullous form, the central portion may be bullous with a marginal ring of vesicles. The lesions come in crops and last for two to three weeks which heal with hypo or hyperpigmentation. Commonly affected sites are the face, dorsal surface of the hand and feet, extensor surfaces of forearm and legs, palms and soles. The mucous membranes are often involved in vesico-bullous form of erythema multiforme.

In severe bullous from (Stevens-Johnson syndrome), extensive bualle and ulcerations develop on the mucous membranes of the mouth, eyes and the genitals and the skin lesions may be maculopapular, vesicular orbullous. The disease is usually associated with marked constitutional symptoms. Systemic involvement may occur affecting the respiratory, renal and alimentary system.

Histologically, the dermal blood vessels are dilated and surrounded by non specific infiltrate. When bullae are present, they are subepidermal. Necrosis of epidermis is seen in severe form.

Treatment

Treatment is rarely needed as the disease is self limiting. Any recognised cause must be eradicated. For milder cases, only symptomic treatment in the form of application of soothing agents such as calamine lotion, is recommended.

Systemic corticosteroids may be prescribed for severe from of erythrema multiforme and a systemic antibiotic should be administered to prevent secondary infections.

11

Disorders of Sebaceous Glands

Sebaceous glands are present all over the body except on the palms, the soles and dorsal surfaces of the hand and foot. They are particularly large and numerous on the scalp, the face, the back and the front of the chest. Each sebaceous gland is composed of multiple lobules of epithelial cells. The duct of each lobules converge towards the main sebaceous duct which normally opens into hair follicle (pilosebaceous unit). Only a small number of sebaceous glands open directly on the surface of the skin (the prepuce, labia minora, eyelids, nipples and lips).

The gland's secretion, sebum, is formed by fatty degeneration of the epithelial cells of the gland. The entire sebaceous cells and its contents are then eliminated into the duct (Holocrine process) and is excreted on to the skin surface through the lumen of the hair follicle. Sebaceous gland activity is under hormonal control. Androgens are the most potent stimulants of sebum production while oestrogens suppress sebaceous gland activity. Sebum contains a complex mixture of lipids i.e., triglycerides, wax esters, squalene, cholestrol ester and cholesterol. The sebum acts as a lubricant and controls moisture loss from the epidermis. Another advantage of sebum is protection of skin from fungal and bacterial infection.

ACNE VULGARIS

Acne vulgaris is a chronic inflammatory disorder of pilosebaceous unit characterized by the development of comedones, papules, nodules and cysts.

Aetio-pathogenesis

Acne predominantly affects adolescents. The peak incidence is between ages 14 and 16 years in girls and 16 and 19 years in boys.

The basic cause of acne is still unknown. It seems to be a multifactorial disease in which interaction of several factors play an important part in the pathogenesis. The primary event may be (a) obstruction of the sebaceous duct due to alteration in the pattern of keratinization within the follicle, (b) abnormal sebum production with excess quantities or altered composition or (c) increased bacterial colonization) proprionibacterium acnes and staphylococcus epidermidis) of pilosebaceous follicles which furnish the lipases responsible for hydrolysis of sebum triglycerides into free fatty acids. All three mechanisms may be involved. Obstruction of duct leads to formation of a comedone, the initial lesion of acne. A comedone can be located either in a closed follicle as a 'white head' consisting of lipid and keratin, or in an open follicle as 'black head' consisting of keratin and lipid with melanin deposition. The continual accumulation of keratin and lipid may lead to rupture of the follicular wall and release of its contents into the surrounding dermis provoking an inflammatory tissue reaction.

Certain factors such as genetic, climate, stress use of drugs and comedogenic chemicals are known to modify acne.

Clinical Features

The disease is characterized by a great variety of lesions which vary from patient to patient but most patients have multiple types of lesions. Various types of lesions are comedones (black or white), papules, pustules, nodules and cysts. There may be post inflammatory hyperpigementation. The common sites are the face, the upper chest, back and the upper arm. In milder form, the comedones predominate the picture and the pustules are relatively infrequent. In severe form, there is preponderance of inflammatory papules, pustules, nodules and cystic lesions. Scarring frequently follows severe type of acne.

Most acne patients have an oily skin with patulous follicular openings. The course of the disease is chronic with frequent remissions and relapses. In majority of the cases, disease tends to subside spontaneously about the age of 25, but may persist indefinitelv.

PLATE I

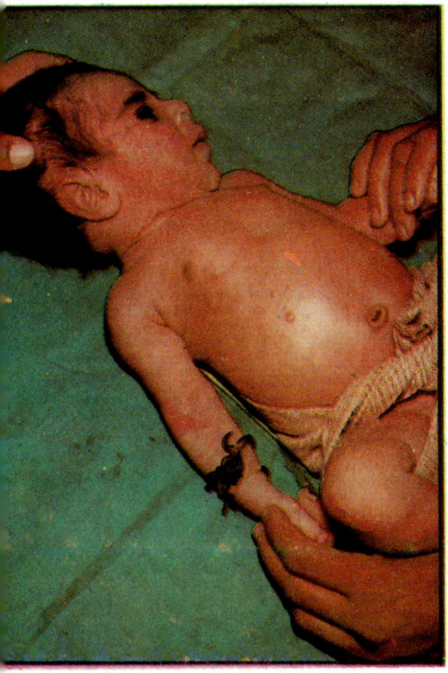

BULLOUS IMPETIGO

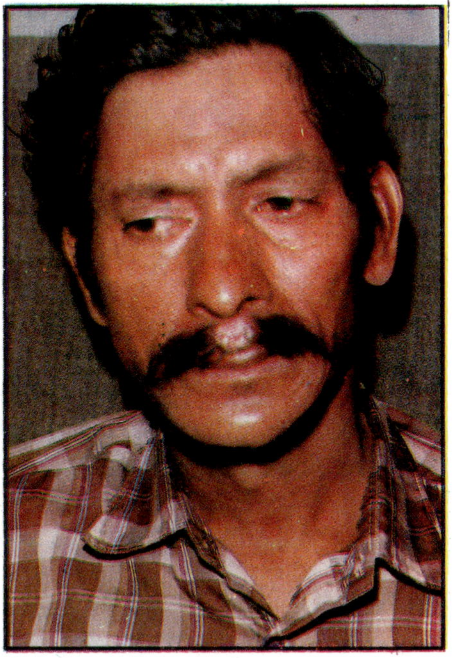

KERION

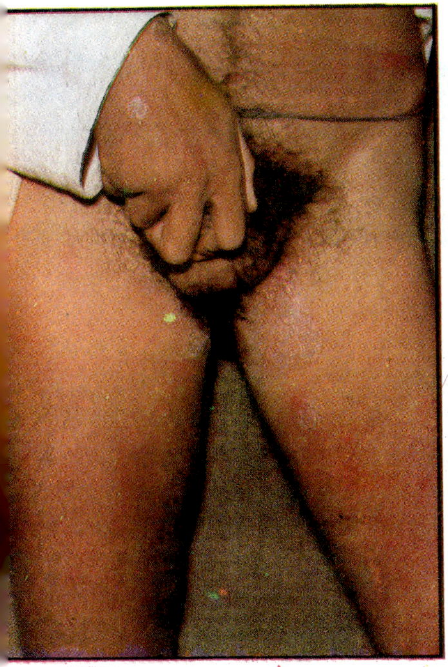

TINEA CRURIS

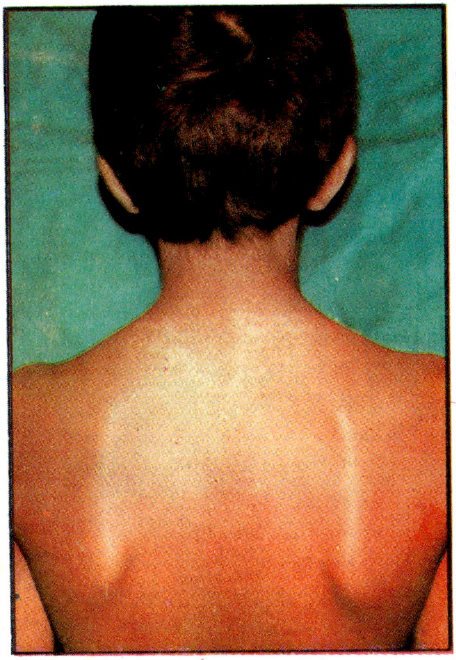

PITYRIASIS VERSICOLOR

PLATE II

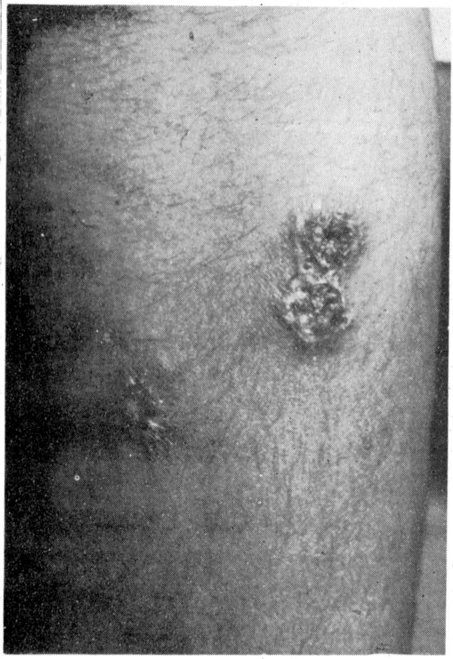

IMPETIGO CONTAGIOSA

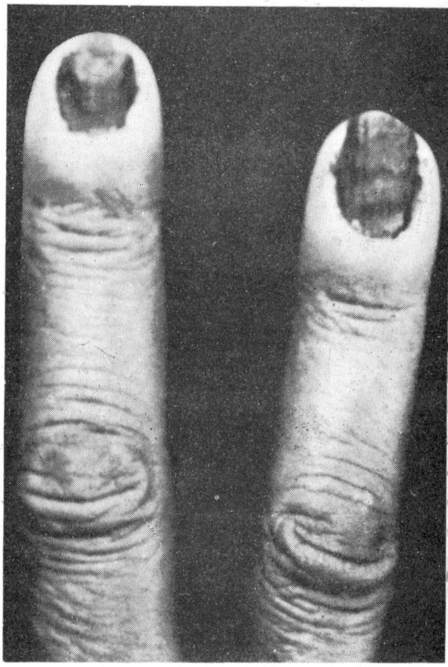

CHRONIC PARONYCHIA

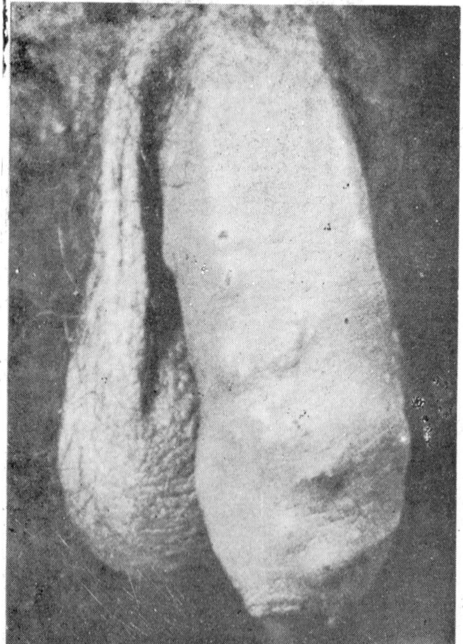

SCABIES

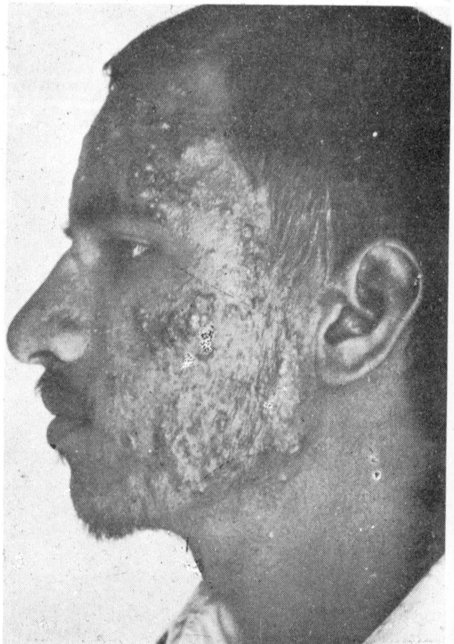

ACNE VULGARIS

PLATE III

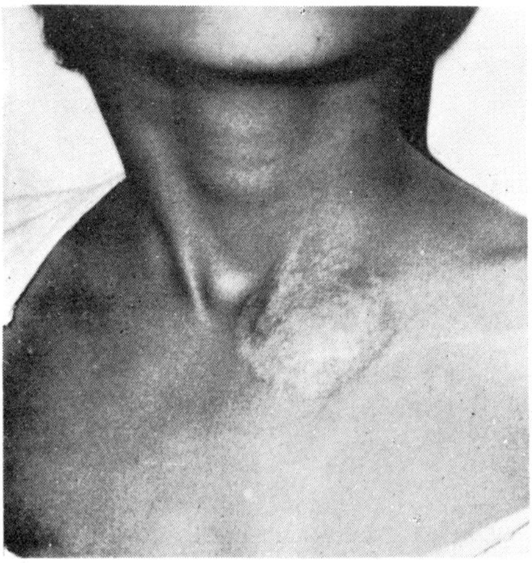

TINEA CORPORIS

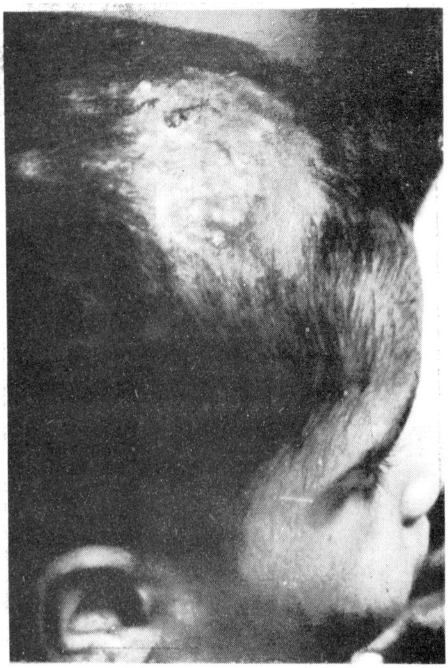

TINEA CAPITIS

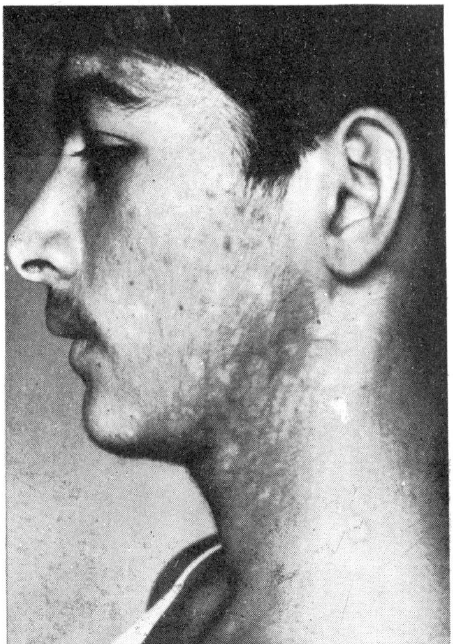

PITYRIASIS VERSICOLOR

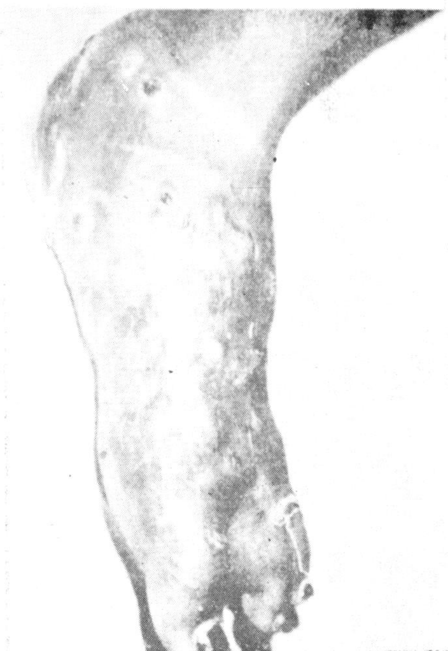

MYCETOMA

PLATE IV

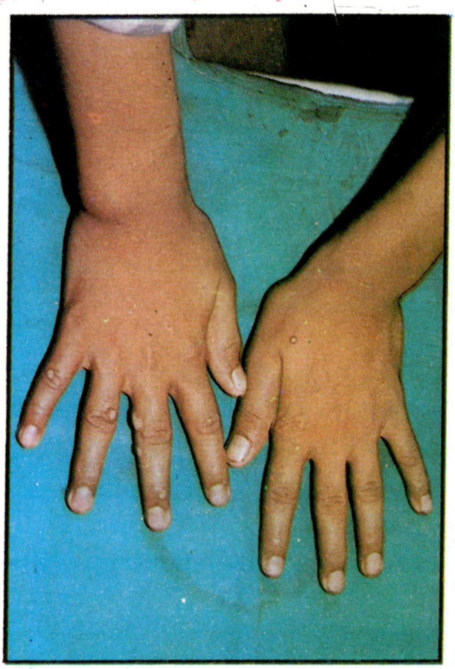

VERRUCA VULGARIS

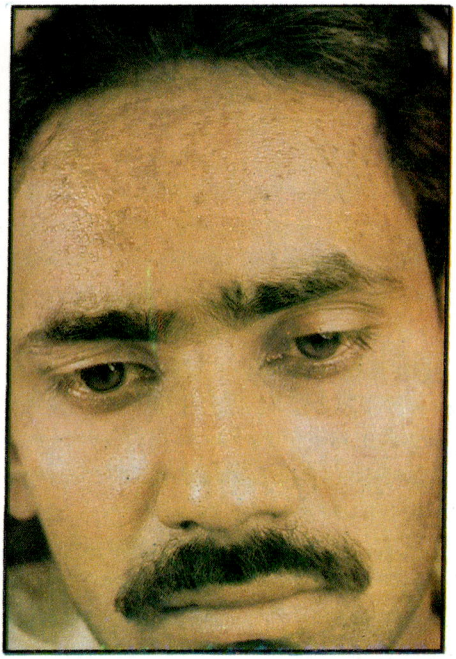

VERRUCA PLANA

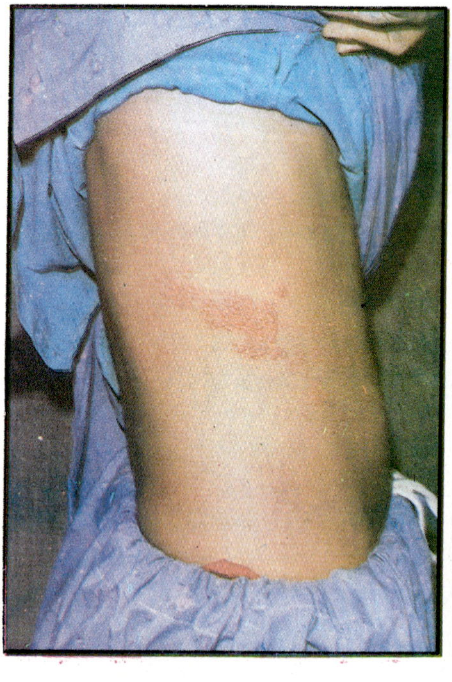

HERPES ZOSTER

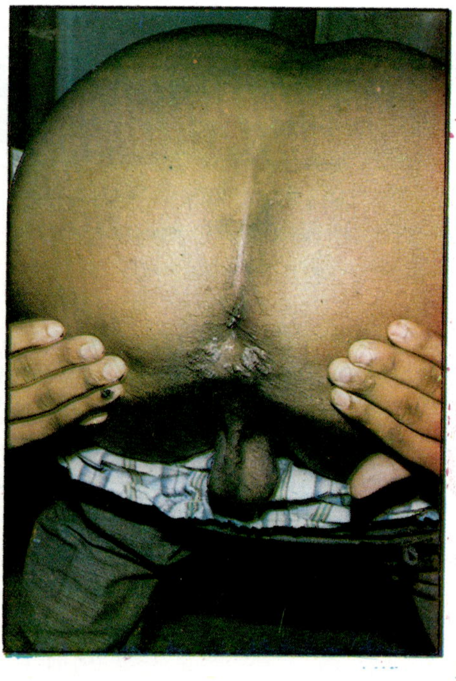

CONDYLOMA ACUMINATA

PLATE V

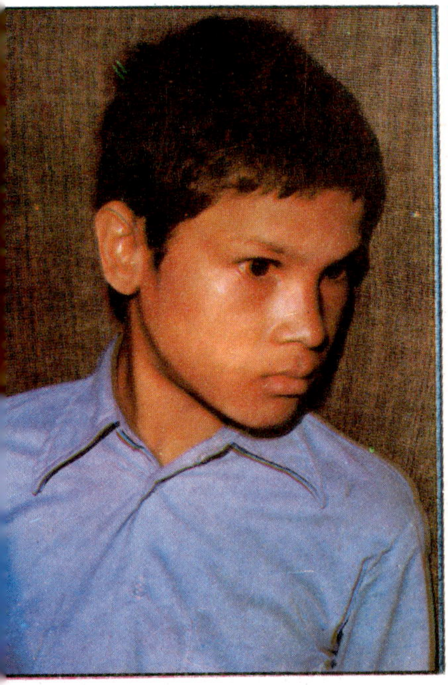

PITYRIASIS ALBA

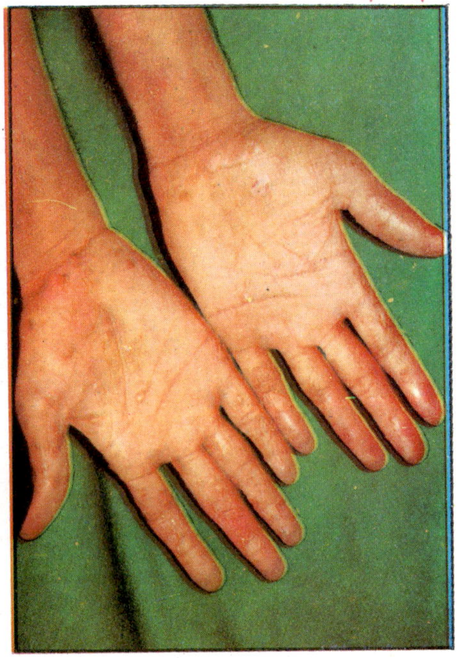

POMPHOLYX

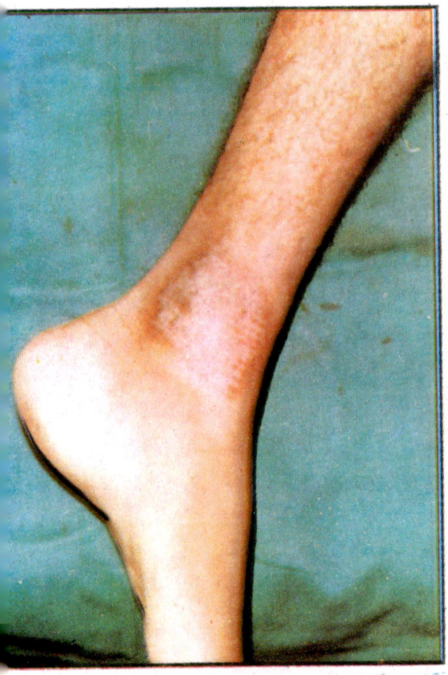

LICHEN SIMPLEX CHRONICUS

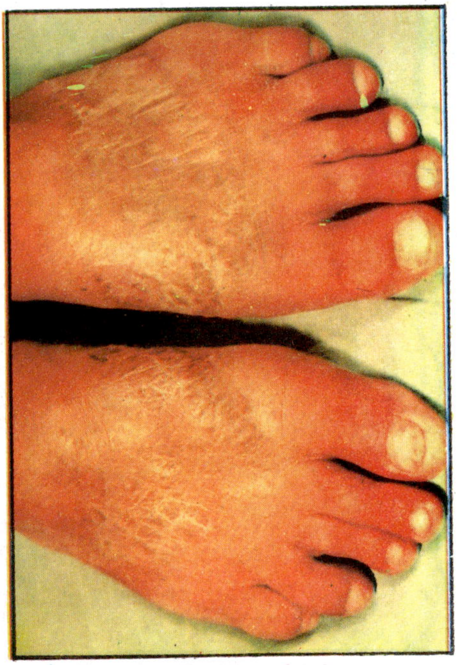

CONTACT DERMATITIS

PLATE VI

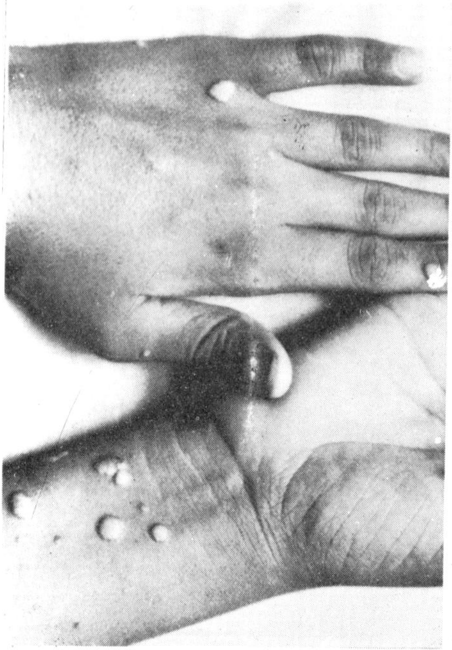

VERRUCA VULGARIS

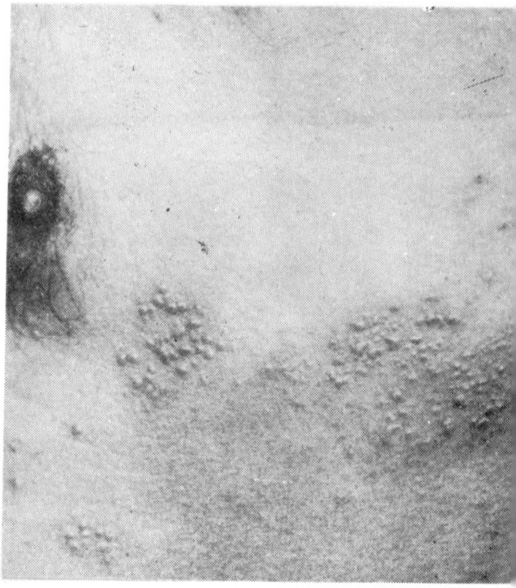

HERPES ZOSTER

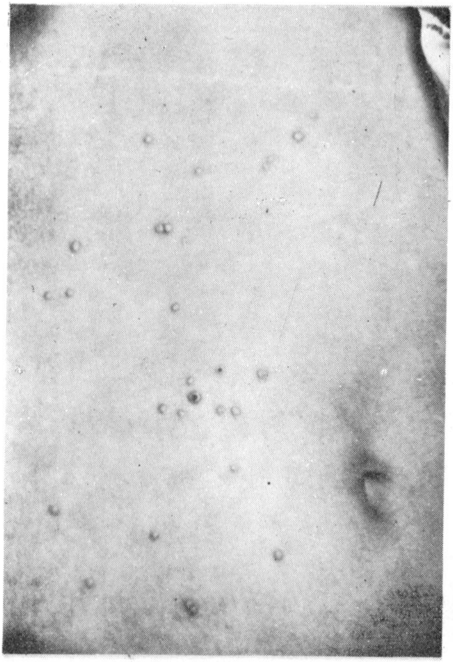

MOLLUSCUM CONTAGIOSUM

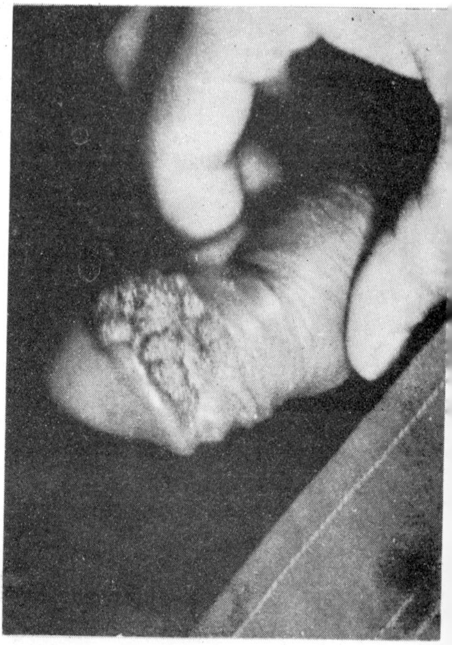

VENEREAL WARTS

PLATE VII

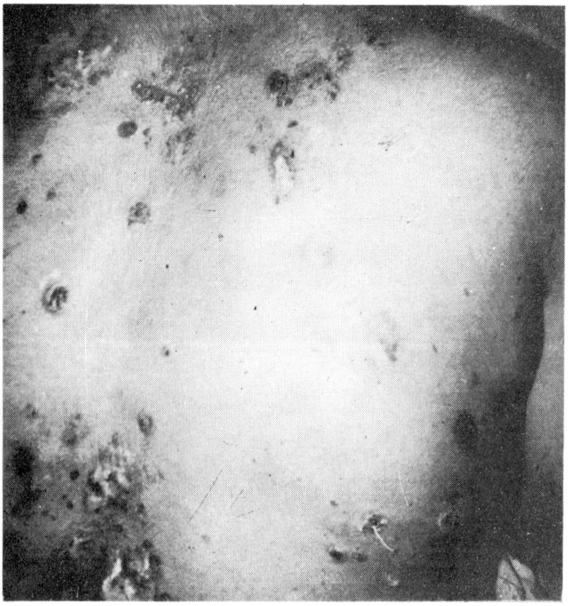

PEMPHIGUS VULGARIS

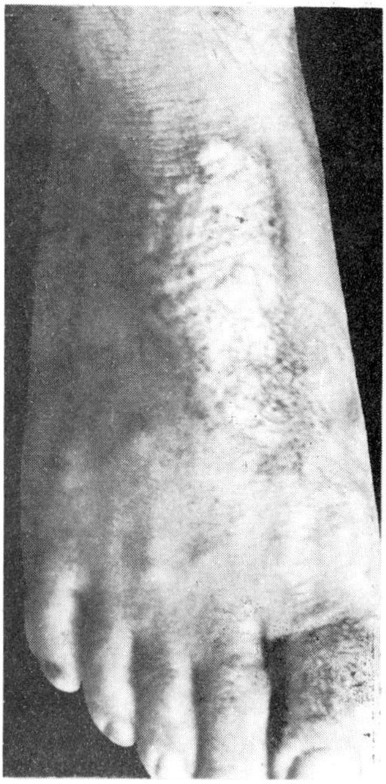

LICHEN SIMPLEX CHRONICUS

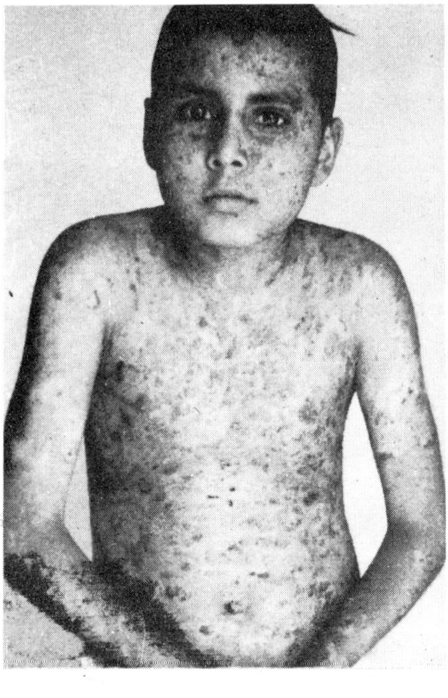

PEMPHIGUS FOLIACEOUS

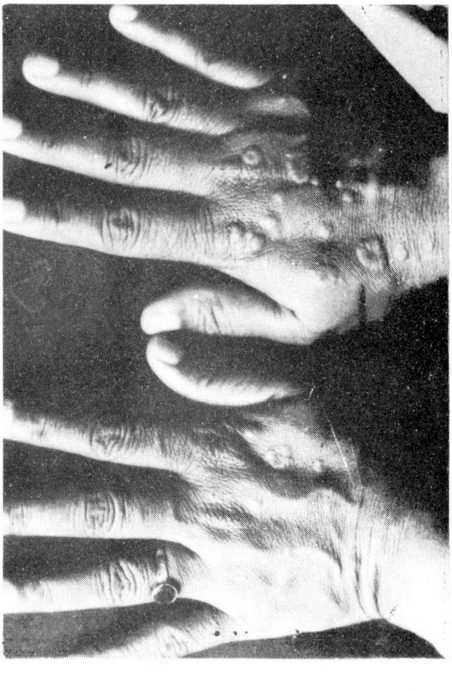

LICHEN PLANUS ACTINICUS

PLATE VIII

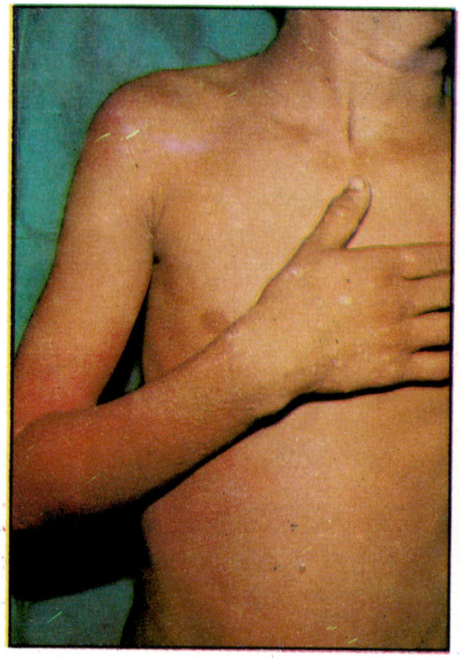

LICHEN PLANUS

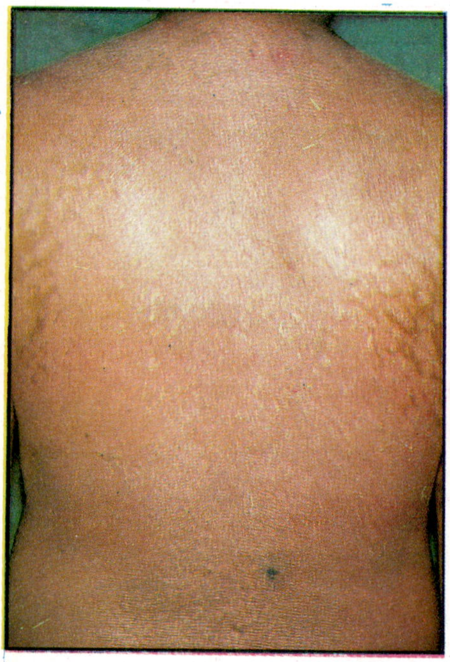

PSORIATIC ERYTHRODERMA

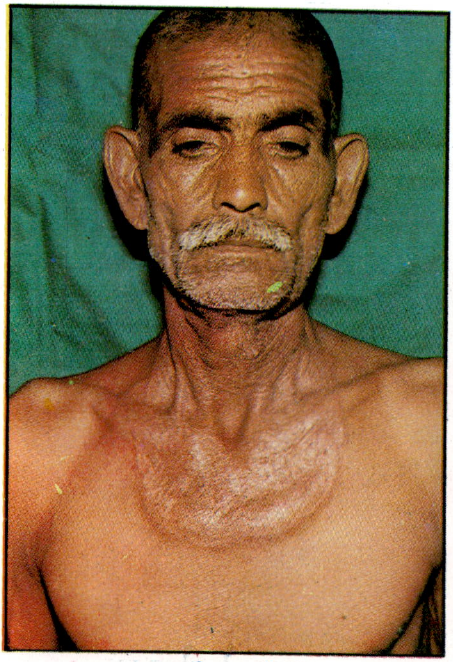

TINEA CORPORIS

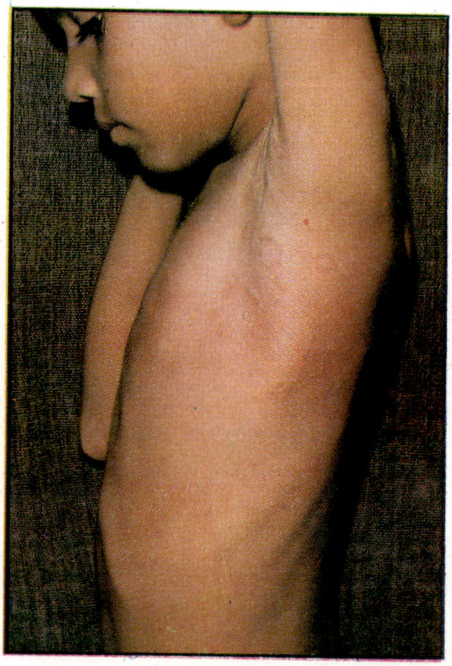

PITYRIASIS ROSEA

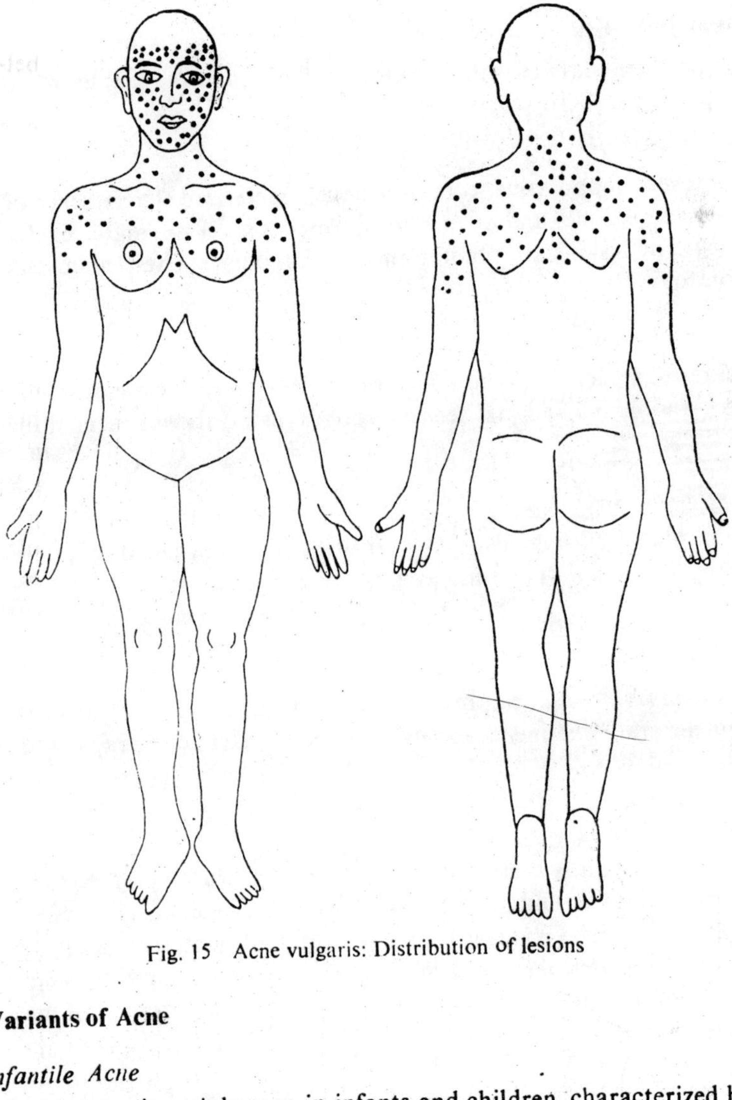

Fig. 15 Acne vulgaris: Distribution of lesions

Variants of Acne

Infantile Acne

Infantile acne is mainly seen in infants and children, characterized by presence of comedones, papules or pustules on the face.

Excoriated Acne

Excoriation dominate in this type of acne, and is largely due to excessive squeezing and picking of acne lesions. This is mainly seen in adolescent girls under emotional stress.

Premenstrual Acne

There is tendency of acne lesions to flare up in the premensturai phase.

Acne Conglobata

It is a severe suppurative form of acne, characterized by presence of comedones, nodules and cysts with burrowing abscesses and irregular scarring. The lesions are situated chiefly on the back, chest, shoulders and buttocks.

Acne Medicamentosa

Certain drugs particularly iodides, bromides, INH, corticosteroids, ACTH, androgens and oral contraceptives can produce acne form eruptions.

Occupational Acne

Many insoluble cutting oils. tars, cosmetics and chlorinated aromatic hydrocarbons can induce acne by external contact.

Treatment

There are several major approaches to treatment of acne vulgaris including general treatment, topical therapy, systemic therapy and physical modalities.

General Treatment

Oiliness of the skin is best controlled by frequent washing of the face with soap and water and to avoid use of greasy cosmetics. No dietery restrictions should be imposed on the patients. Psychiatric counselling may be required in severe cases of acne with emotional upset. Patients should be advised to avoid further squeezing or manipulation of the lesions.

Topical Therapy

This is designed to produce peeling of the skin, restore normal keratinization and produce a bactericidal action. Common peeling agents are sulphur (3-5%), resorcin (3-5%), benzyl peroxide (5-10%) and retinoic acid (0.025-0.1%). Peeling agents should be applied once or twice a day, taking care to avoid excessive irritation.

Topical antibiotics include erythromycin (1-2%), clindamycin (1-2%) and benzyl peroxide (5-10%). **Benzyl peroxide has bacterio-**

static properties in addition to its action as a peeling agent. Comedones may be expressed with a comedo-extractor and cyst should be drained and injected with corticosteroids.

Systemic Therapy

The antibiotics such as tetracycline, erythromycin, clindamymin and cotrimoxazole are most commonly used in the treatment of acne vulgaris. Tetracycline is the treatment of choice for moderate to severe acne and is given in the dosage of 250 mg three to four times daily with a gradual reduction to a maintenance dose of 250 mg once a day for several months. Recently, oral retinoids (isotretinoin) has been found to be very effective drug in the management of severe form of acne, especially nodulocystic acne and conglobata.

Anti-androgens like cyproterone acetate and spironolactone are also beneficial in treatment of acne. Females with recalcitrant and severe type of acne usually require oestrogens either in the form of oral contraceptives or in combination with antiandrogens.

Physical Modalities

Physical measures include exposure to ultraviolet light, irradiation and exfoliation with carbon dioxide snow (cryotherapy). Dermabrasions may be required for treatment of depressed scars.

ROSACEA

Rosacea is a chronic disease of unknown cause, characterized by redness with dilated blood vessels (Telangiectasia) and oedematous papules and pustules, limited to the central facial area. It is aggravated by heat, sunlight, spicy foods, hot drinks and alcohol. It mainly affects middle aged females. In males, the nose may become enlarged and lobulated (Rhinophyma). Occasionally rosacea is accompanied by blephritis, conjunctivitis and keratits.

Rosacea may be distinguished from acne vulgaris by the absence of comedones and scars.

Treatment

Oral tetracycline in dosage of 250 mg two to three times a day for 1-2 weeks, then once daily for a few months, is effective. Topically, hydrocortisone (1%) and acne peeling agents have also been used.

12

Disorders of Hair

Hair is found on almost every part of the body except on the palms, the soles, dorsum of the terminal phalanges of the digits, the glans penis and the mucocutaneous junctions. There are three main types of hair:

1. Lanugo hair is short, soft, fine and lightly pigmented, usually present in foetus, (2) Vellus hair is fine and lightly pigmented which covers the body of the children and young adults, (3) Terminal hair is long, coarse and pigmented, present on the scalp, the eye brows and the eye lashes prepubertally and subsequently in the axillary and pubic region as 'secondary sexual hair'.

Hair follicle and its hair in longitudinal section can be divided into three segments: (1) infundibulum, which extend from follicular orifice above to the entrance of sebaceous gland below, (2) Isthmus, which extend from the entrance of sebaceous duct above to insertion of the arrector pilorum muscle below and (3) inferior segment, which extend from the insertion of the arrector pilorum muscle to the base of the follicle.

Each hair follicle consists of a dermal hair papilla, the hair matrix, the hair, the inner root sheath and the outer root sheath. The hair matrix is the site of intense mitotic activity, which results in the formation of the hair shaft. From outside inward, each hair shaft consists of hair cuticle, cortex and medulla.

The growth of the hair is cyclical. Three phases of life cycle are: (1) anagen (the growing phase), the hair continues to increase in length at a rate of approximately 1 cm per month but it varies with the site of the follicle (approximately 3 years in the scalp) and the age of the subject, (2) catagen (the involuting phase), the follicular mitotic activity ceases and follicle begins to shrink (approximately lasting

.or 3 weeks) and (3) telogen (resting phase) last for 3 months. The old shrunked hair is shed at the end of telogen phase and new hair regrow around the old dermal papilla.

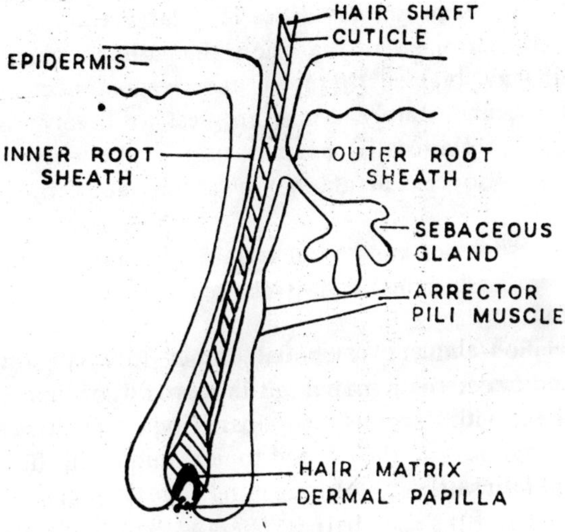

Fig. 16 Vertical section of hair follicle in digrammatic form

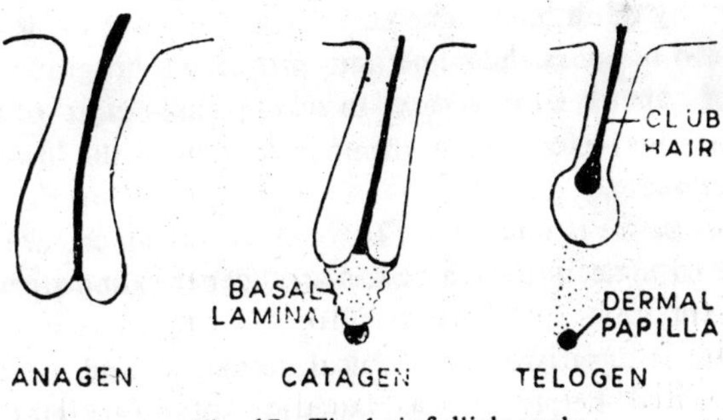

Fig. 17 The hair follicle cycle

ALOPECIA (HAIR LOSS)

The alopecias can be ciassified as: (1) Non-cicatricial and (2) Cicatricial.

Non-Cicatracial Alopecia

This is a non-scarring alopecia where the hair follicles are retained and the hair loss is potentially reversible.

Alopecia Areata

This is a common condition mainly affecting children and young adults. The disease is characterized by asymptomatic, circuiar or oval, smooth patches of complete loss of hair on the scalp, the beard or elsewhere. There is no evidence of inflammation, scarring or atrophy. On the periphery of the lesion, the pathognomonic exclamation mark hair may be seen. In most cases, spontaneous recovery and regrowth occurs. Rarely, it may progress to involve all the hair of the scalp (alopecia totalis) and even hair of the whole body (alopecia universalis). Alopecia areata may be accompanied by pitting of nail plate.

Exact cause is not known but certain factors such as genetic, immunological, endo crinal and psychological have been incriminated in its aetiology.

No specific treatment is available, but topical, intralesional and systemic corticosteroids may result in regrowth of hair. Relapses may occur after withdrawl of corticosteriods. Dinitrochlorobenzene (DNCB) scnsitization, PUVA and topical minoxidil have been used with variable results.

Male Pattern Alopecia

This is a progressive, symmetric, diffuse loss of terminal hair from the scalp affecting adult male. The hair loss usually begins, with recession of the fronto temporal hair line and progresses to gradual thinning and loss of hair over the vertex. In severe cases most of the hair on the scalp are lost except for a thin rim of hair on the lower sides and back of the scalp.

The exact cause is unknown. Three factors which are known to predispose to male pattern alopecia are: genetic, androgens, and age of the patient.

Treatment is unsatisfatory. Topical minoxidil and oestrogen preparation may be helpful. Transplantation of punch grafts from the hairy occiput to the bald area is helpful in selected cases.

Diffuse Alopecia

The condition is characterized by diffuse shedding of scalp hair, mainly affecting young females. The patient looses 100-200 hair per day depending upon the severity of the disease. The cause is usually detectable in history and occur about three months before the hair begin to fall.

It is most often precipitated by a prolonged fever, deblitating disease, pregancy, treatment with certain drugs (cytotoxic, thalium and heparin), surgical shock or severe emotional stress.

Prognosis is uniformally good and the hair regrow to its former state in due course of time.

No treatment is required except for ascertaining the cause and reassuring the patient.

Cicatricial Alopecia

Cicatracial alopecia is a scarring type of alopecia in which the hair follicles are destroyed and the hair loss is therefore, irreversible. The skin is usually atrophic or scarred. Important causes of cicatricial alopecia are: (1) physical trauma (burn, x-ray irradiation and long term traction on the hair), (2) fungal infections (kerion and favus), (3) bacterial infections (lupus valgaris, carbuncle, folliculitis decalvans), (4) viral infections (herpes zoster) and (5) cutaneous diseases (pseudoplade, follicular lichen planus, lupus erythematosus and scleroderma).

HIRSUTISM AND HYPERTRICHOSIS

Hirsutism is characterized by an excessive growth of terminal hair in women on androgen dependent areas of the body (upper lip, chin, centre of the chest, abdomen and anterior aspects of the thighs). It may be accompanied by virilism, which consist of hypertrophy of clitoris, deepening of the voice, acne, increase in muscular mass, breast involution and recession of fronto-temporal hair line. Different causes of hirsutism are divided into two main groups:

(1) Endocrinal causes: Polycystic ovary, congenital adrenal hyperplasia, adrenal adenoma and hilus cell tumour, (2) Non endocrinal causes: Racial, familial, idiopathic and certain drugs (phenytoin, minoxidil, androgen and corticosteroid).

Hypertrichosis is an increase in hair growth which is not androgen dependent and is most often of nonendocrine origin.

Treatment

Treatment consists of a three pronged attack using cosmetic methods (waxing, bleaching, use of depilatory cream and electrolysis), suppressive therapy (Dexamethasone and oral contraceptives) and peripheral androgen blockers (spironolactone and cyproterone acetate).

13

Disorders of the Nails

Each nail consists of a hard nail plate which emerges from the matrix. Its lateral and proximal borders are overlapped by lateral and proximal nail folds. A whitish, crescent shaped zone just distal to proximal nail fold is termed as 'Lunula'. The 'Cuticle' is an extension of the horny layer of the epidermis on to the nail plate whlch normally seals off the potential space in the nail fold. The skin underlying the free end of the nail is referred to as the 'Hyponychium' which is continuous with the skin on the tip of the finger. Nail bed is the area which extends from lunula to hyponychium.

Nail bed and matrix is supplied by paired digital arteries. The finger nails grow much faster than the toe nails. Abnormalities of nails can be discussed under two main groups:

NAIL DYSTROPHIES

1. Onycholysis

This is a painless separation of the nail plate from the nail bed at its distal end. The seperated area of the nail plate looks pale due to loss of light reflexion from the nail bed. Common causes of onycholysis are trauma, psoriasis, eczema, fungal infection, thyroid disorders, yellow nail syndrome, heriditary, certain drugs like dimethyl-chlortetracycline and nail hardeners.

2. Pterygium

This is a fusion of dorsal nail fold and nail matix with partial loss of nail plate. This is largely due to destruction of nail matrix. The

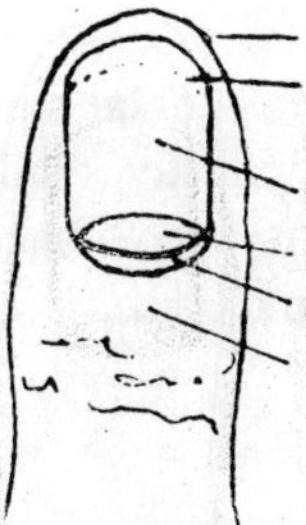

Fig. 18 The nail

common causes of ptrerygium are impaired circulation, lichen planus and rarely idiopathic.

3. Onychogryphosis

This is an acquired thickening of the nail which usually becomes curved. It is often secondary to trauma.

4. Koilonychia

In this condition, there is spoon shaped depression of the nail plate which is often associated with iron deficiency anaemia but in some cases it may be familial.

5. Beau's Lines

These are the transvese depression in the nails as a result of decrease in the size of nail matrix and are mainly due to coronary disorders, viral diseases, zinc deficiency and chronic dermatitis like exfoliative dermatitis.

6. Pitting

Pits are nothing but small depressions in the nail plate. They are due to abnormal keratinization in the matrix resulting into formation of small areas of weak keratin which is then shed and forms pits. Pits usually occur in psoriasis, alopecia areata and rarely in eczema and lichen planus.

7. Clubbing

It is the loss of normal angle between dorsal nail fold and the nail. The common causes are: Chronic suppurative lung diseases, bronchogenic carcinoma, cyanotic heart disease, Subacute bacterial endocarditis, ulcerative colitis and cirrhosis.

8. Pigmentation

White nails are seen in leukonychia which may be total or partial. The total leuconychia is usually a genetic disorder while the partial whitening is either spontaneons or due to minor trauma. White nails are also seen in cirrhosis of liver, chronic renal failure and fungal infection. A blue black nail is seen in subungual haematoma and prolonged therapy with chloroquine. Yellow nails are seen in yellow nail syndrome, psoriasis, fungal infections and due to tetracyline. Small brown linear streaks in the nail plate may be due to splinter haemorrhages.

9. Lamellar Dystrophy

This is a splitting of the tips of the nails into layers. The causes are repeated wetting of the hands, use of nail cosmetics, iron deficiency anaemia and impaired peripheral circulation.

10. Ridging

These may be longitudinal or transverse which may be idiopathic or secondary to many dermatosis such as psoriasis, fungal infections, eczemas, lichen planus etc.

DISEASES OF THE NAIL FOLD

1. Chronic Paronychia

Chronic paronychia is an infection of the nail fold caused by anaerobic organisms and candida. It is usually seen in young and middle aged women, whose hands are constantly in water. Predisposing causes also include poor peripheral circulation, diabetes and certain occupations like kitchen, laundary and canteen workers etc.

The nail fold becomes red, tender and swollen and it separates from the plate resulting in a space. Gentle pressure often causes a bead of pus to exude from beneath the nail fold. As the condition persists, the emerging nail plate often becomes discoloured and may show transverse ridging.

Treatment

Treatment consists of encouraging the patient to keep the hands as dry as possible. Local application with 1% aqueous solution of gentian violet, nystatin ointment. miconazole or clotrimozole lotion may be helpful.

2. Ingrowing Toe Nails

Improper cutting of the nail plate results into formation of spicules of nail at the edges of the nail plate which penetrate into the soft tissue of the lateral fold causing pain, infection and formation of granulation tissue. Tight fitted shoes may also contribute in causation of this disorder. The great toe is most commonly affected.

Treatment

The contributing factors like wearing of tight fitted shoes and improper cutting of nail plate should be avoided. The nail plate should be cut straight across. Milder cases require application of Trichloroacetic acid or silver nitrate solution to cauterize the granulation tissue. In some cases, avulsion of nail plate may be indicated under local anaesthesia. Systemic antibiotics may be required in presence of secondary bacterial infections.

14

Disorders of Sweat Glands

Sweat glands are of two types, eccrine and apocrine. Eccrine glands are true sweat glands distributed all over the skin except at mucocutaneous junctions and are most highly concentrated on the palms, soles, axillae and forehead. Each eccrine sweat gland consists of a coiled secretory part, coiled dermal duct, straight dermal duct and a spiral intraepidermal duct. These glands are innervated by unmyelinated cholinergic sympathetic fibers. The eccrine sweet is an odourless, colourless, hypotonic solution, which flows on to the skin surface and cools the body by evoporation.

Apocrine glands occur in the axillae, areolae, umbilicus and anogential region. Each apocrine gland consists of a coiled secretary part and a straight excretory duct. Apocrine glands produce secretion by the process of pinching off parts of the secretory cells. The apocrine secretion is odourless but subsequent bacterial decomposition on the skin surface gives a characteristic odour. The glands have no apparent functions in the human beings.

DISORDERS OF ECCRINE SWEAT GLANDS

Hyperhidrosis

Hyperhidrosis can be defined as an increased production of sweat which may be generalized or localized. The different stimuli which can cause excessive sweat production are gustatory (spicy foods), thermal or emotional. This disorder usually begins around puberty and improves at the age of 25. Hyperhidrosis of feet predisposes patient to tinea pedis and plantar warts. Topical application of aluminium salts, formalin soaks (2-5%), ingestion of anticholinergic and tranquilizers, iontophoresis and surgical excision of axillary sweat glands have all been tried with variable results.

Hypohidrosis and Anhidrosis

Hypohidrosis can be defined as a decrease secretion of sweat, even on appropriate stimuli. Anhidrosis is complete absence of sweating in response to appropriate stimuli. The common causes are congenital ectodermal dysplasias, ichthyosis, leprosy, diabetes, Horner's syndrome, erythroderma and miliaria.

Miliaria

Miliaria is due to blockage of the sweat duct usually caused by excessive heat and humidity. There are three types of miliaria: (1) miliaria crystallina, (2) miliaria rubra and (3) miliaria profundus.

Miliaria crystallina results from blockage of the mouth of the sweat duct (sweat pore) and is characterized by appearance of asymptomatic, tiny shiny vesicles on normal looking skin.

Miliaria-rubra (prickly heat) is due to blockage of sweat duct in its intraepidermal part and is characterized by appearance of small grouped papules or papulovesicles surrounded by erythema. It produces intense pruritus. The common sites of affection are the trunk and neck.

Miliaria profounda occurs when the blockage of the sweat duct is at the dermo-epidermal junction. The lesions are skin coloured papules mainly seen on the trunk and the extremities.

Treatment of miliaria should be directed toward prevention of excessive sweating and avoidance of soap, hot water and irritants. In cases with severe itching, local application of calamine lotion is recommended and may be supplemented with oral antihistamines. Ascorbic acid 1 gm daily may be of prophylactic value.

DISORDERS OF APOCRINE GLANDS

Hidradenitis Suppurativa

This is a chronic suppurative and cicatricial disease of the apocrine glands affecting the axillae or anogenital regions. The lesions are multiple, erythematous, tender swellings which turn into fluctuating masses. The lesions may coalesce and discharging through multiple sinuses. The lesions heal with fibrosis and scarring. Systemic antibiotoics are effective in early cases. In severe cases surgical excision and skin grafting of the affected part may be required.

Bromhidrosis

Bromhidrosis is a disease in which there is excessive or abnormal skin odour and is generally confined to axillae (apocrine bromhidrosis) or feet (eccrine bromhidrosis). It usually results from hyperhidrosis and bacterial decomposition of sweat. Treatment consists of frequent washing and application of antibacterial agents.

Chromhidrosis

Chromhidrosis is secretion of coloured sweat. True eccrine chromhidrosis is very uncommon and when present it is usually due to ingestion of drugs and dyes. Apocrine chromhidrosis is usually seen in the axillae and on the face. The most common colour is yellow, blue or green and pigment responsible is usually lipofuscin.

Treatment is unsatisfactory. The glands may be removed surgically.

Fox Fordyce Disease

In fox fordyce disease, the lesion are pruritic, skin coloured, dome shaped papules affecting the axillae, pubis and mammary region. It results from obstruction and rupture of intraepidermal portion of the duct of affected apocrine gland. This disease occurs mainly in adult women at or shortly after puberty.

Treatment is unsatisfactory. Topical and intralesional corticosteroids, oral contraceptives and radiotherapy have all been tried with variable results. Surgical excision may be required in severe cases.

15

Disorders of Pigmentation

Melanin is an inert pigment which is synthesized from tyrosine in specialized cytoplasmic organelles called 'Melanosomes' which are numerous in melanocytes. Melanocytes contain enzymes which convert tyrosine into melanin in the following manner:

$$\text{Tyrosine} \xrightarrow[\text{(Slow oxidation)}]{\text{Tyrosinase}} \text{Dihydroxyphenylalanine (L-dopa)}$$

$$\text{Melanin} \leftarrow \text{Dopaquinone} \xleftarrow[\text{(Fast oxidation)}]{\text{Tyrosinase}} \text{(L-dopa)}$$

Fully melanisied melanosomes are transferred to the adjacent keratinocytes via dendrities of melanocytes. The quantity of melanin in the skin varies from individual to individual, and race to race. Melanin production is influenced by many factors like genetic, hormonal, physical and chemical.

Disorders of melanin pigmentation may be based on an increase in amount (Hypermelanosis), a decrease in amount (Hypomelanosis) or complete absence of pigment (Amelanotic).

HYPERMELANOSIS

Various causes of hypermelanosis are listed in Table 1.

TABLE 1

(A) *Genetic disorders*:	(B) *Endocrinal disorders*:
Freckles	Addison's disease
Lentigenes	Hyperthyroidism
Peutz Jeghar syndrome	Cushing's syndrome
Incontenentia pigmenti	ACTH therapy
Xeroderma pigmentosum	Melasma
Neurofibromatosis	

(C) *Drugs*:
Phenothiazines
Antimalarials
Antiepileptics
Antimitotic
Arsenic
Psoralen

(D) *Systemic disorders*:
Chronic infections like malaria and kala azar
Lymphoma
Collagen disorders
Renal failure
Anaemia
Liver diseases
Vitamin A, B_{12} and folate deficiency
Malabsorption syndrome
Pellagra
Amyloidosis
Porphyria

(E) *Post inflammatory*:
Eczema
Lichen planus

(F) *Physical agents*:
Ultraviolet rays
Ionizing radiation

Freckles

Freckles are characterized by small, light, brown macules on the sun exposed areas of the skin, often seen in fair skinned individuals. They appear usually in childhood. There is no increase in the number of the melanocytes, but the melanosomes are abnormally long and are more active than those in the surrounding skin and therefore the freckles darken on sun exposure. Treatment consists mainly of protection of skin from sun exposure either by avoidance of sunlight or by use of sun screens.

Lentigenes

Lentigenes are brown macules which result from an increase in epidermal melanocytes. They may occur on all parts of the body, especially the covered parts. They are darker than freckles and are not affected by exposure to sunlight. No treatment is required except for cosmetic reasons. Topical retinoic acid or liquid nitrogen may be helpful.

Melasma (Chloasma)

This is a common condition, characterized by well defined, brown pigmented patches on the cheek, forehead, and the upper lip. The lesions are usually symmetrical. It is mainly seen in females, occuring during pregnancy and in those who are on oral contraceptives. Lesions may fade in post partum period or after discontinuation of oral contraceptive but often persist.

Treatment consists of avoidance of sun exposure and use of sun screens like paraaminobenzoic acid (5-10%). Topical application of 2-5% hydroquinone with 0.1% retinoic acid and 0.025% triamcinolone acetate may be useful.

HYPOMELANOSIS

Various causes of hypomelanosis are listed in Table 2.

TABLE 2

(A) *Genetic factors*:	(B) *Endocrinal factors*:
Vitiligo	Hypopituitarism
Plebaldism	Addison's disease
Albinism	Hyperthyroidism
Phenylketonuria	
(C) *Nutritional factors*:	(D) *Chemicals*:
Chronic protein deficiency	Monobenzyl ether of hydroquinone
Vit. B_{12} deficiency	Topical steroid
	Retinoic acid
(E) *Post inflammatory and infections*:	(F) *Tumours*:
Eczema	Halo naevus
Psoriasis	Malignant melanoma
Leprosy	
Pityriasis versicolor	
Pityriasis alba	

Vitiligo

Vitiligo is a common, acquired, patchy depigmentation or hypopigmentation of the skin. It is probably an autoimmune disease. Evidence for this view is largely due to its association with other autoimmune disorders like diabetes, alopecia areata, pernicious anaemia etc. Genetic predisposition is also seen in some cases. Other theories suggested for the aetiology of vitiligo are self destruction of melanocytes and neurogenic theory.

Clinical Features

Most patients with vitiligo have no symptoms apart from a cosmetic disability and great social embarrassment. The lesions are depigmented or hypopigmented macules and patches of varying sizes and shapes with distinct margin. Lesions may be discrete or confluent. The hair in the lesions may be depigmented. The distribution of the lesions is usually symmetrical but may be focal or segmental. The most commonly affected sites are the face, the dorsum of the hand, the axillae, the groin, knee, ankle and feet. Mucosal involvement is not uncommon. The depigmentation or hypopigmentation may occur at the site of trauma (Koebner phenomenon). The disease can begin at any age but usually the onset is in young adults. Both sexes are equally affected.

The course of the disease is very variable. Majority of the patients have a progressive involvement of the skin over a period of several months.

Treatment

Treatment of vitiligo is not satisfactory. Trimethylpsoralen and 8-methoxypsoralen have been used orally or topically and followed by exposure to long ultraviolet rays (320-400 mm) from sunlight or artificial sources.

The patient is asked to take psoralen in a dosage of 0.6 mg/kg body weight, 2 hours before graded exposure to either sunlight or artificial long wave ultravoilet light. The frequency of treatment should be at least for 2-3 times a week.

Topical use of psoralen is only recommended for small localized lesions. The lesions are painted with 8-methoxypsoralen lotion followed by exposure to sunlight or artificial long ultraviolet light after 30-45 minutes. To start with, sun exposure is given only for 1-2 minutes which should be increased cautiously to a maximum of 5-10 minutes.

Topical corticosteroid preparations are also found to be effective. Refractory lesions on the exposed parts may need cosmetic masking agent e.g. cover mark and protection from sunlight.

Monobenzyl ether of hydroquinone (10-20%) should be applied in the patients with extensive vitiligo in order to bleach away the remaining pigmented skin.

Piebaldism

Piebaldism is inherited as an autosomal dominant tract and is characterized by congenital, depigmented patches of skin often associated with white forelock of hair. Patches usually remain unchanged throughout life and occur commonly on scalp and forehead but may also occur on the upper chest, abdomen and limbs.

Albinism

Albinism is an autosomal recessive condition in which there is a complete absence of melanin in the skin, hair and eyes. It is due to a defect in the biosynthesis of tyrosinase. Patients have fair skin and blonde hair. They commonly have poor visual acuity, marked photophobia and nystagmus. Albinos are more prone to get skin cancers because of their poor protection from damaging effects of sunlight.

16

Tuberculosis of Skin

Tuberculosis of skin is commonly seen in tropical and developing countries and is caused by Mycobacterium tuberculosis. Tubercle bacilli reach the skin through exogenous inoculation, by haematogenous route or by contiguous spread from neighbouring areas. The clinical picture depends upon the method of cutaneous inoculation and the immunological status of the patient. The common clinical form of tuberculosis of skin are: tubercular chancre, lupus vulgaris, tuberculosis verrucosa cutis and scrofuloderma.

Tubercular Chancre

This is a manifestation of primary cutaneous tuberculosis which occurs in a patient without previous infection and no immunity. The lesion consists of a nodule which soon breaks down forming indolent ulcer with undermined edges. There is associated enlargement of regional lymph nodes. The ulcer heals spontaneously leaving a scar.

Lupus Vulgaris

Lupus vulgaris develops in previously infected individuals with good immunity. The source of infection may be from previous skin inoculation at the same site, from direct extension from underlying focus, or from haematogenous spread.

Initial lesion is a small brownish papule which gradually enlarges. The well formed lesion is characterized by a plaque with scattered pin head size, translucent, reddish brown skin colour papules or nodules (apple jelly nodules). Usually, there is peripheral extension and central healing with scarring. Recurrences of lupus vulgaris may occur in the scar tissue. Other clinical forms of lupus vulgaris may be ulcerative, vegetative, mutilating or mixed forms. The sites of predilection are the nose, cheeks, ear lobes, buttocks, and rarely, the trunk.

Tuberculosis Verrucosa Cutis (TVC)

TVC occurs in previously infected individuals with high degree of immunity, and may be from infected sputum or as a result of occupational handling of infected material. The initial lesion is a small reddish brown warty papule which gradually enlarges and produces a warty hyperkeratotic plaque, with a serpiginous outline. The centre of the lesion may involute leaving a atrophic scar. Sites mostly affected are the hands, feet, knees, ankles and buttocks. The course of the disease is chronic lasting months or years.

Scrofuloderma

This form of cutaneous tuberculosis results from direct extension of infection from underlying tuberculous focus i.e. infected lymph glands, muscles or bones. The patient's immunity is poor or moderate. It usually begins as one or few non tender, bluish red nodules which break down to form ulcers with irregular undermined bluish borders. Untreated scrofuloderma will last for years and heal with disfiguring scars.

Diagnosis of Tuberculosis

Diagnosis of tuberculosis mainly depends on the clinical examination and the laboratory investigations. The laboratory investigations include demonstration of bacilli in smears of biopsy material, culture and inoculation of Gyinea pigs with material from the lesions. Histopathologically, there is tuberculoid granuloma with epitheloid and langhan's giant cells. Caseation may be present.

Treatment

The drugs used for treatment of tuberculosis are isoniazid (INH), streptomycin, rifampicin and ethambutol. Two or three drugs should always be administered simultaneously. The treatment should be continued until all signs of activity have been suppressed for at least six months.

17

Urticaria

Urticaria is a common vascular reaction pattern characterized by dermal swelling due to vasodilatation and increased vascular permeability. Clinically, it is manifested as intensely itchy, erythematous or pale, oedematous swelling which is evanescent in nature.

Mechanism

It is mainly due to local increase of permeability of the capillaries and the small venules. Histamine, which is derived from mast cell, is an important mediator. Kinins, prostaglandins, fibrinolysin system and complements are other important mediators.

Urticaria can be produced by wide variety of immunological and non-immunological (Physical, chemical, drugs) stimuli.

Provoking Causes

Aero-allergens
Blood products and Bites (insects)
Contactants
Drugs
Endogenons diseases
Foods
Genetic diseases
PHysical urticaria
Infections/Infestations and Idiopathic

Aero-allergens

Important aero-allergens are pollens, housedust, feathers, spores etc.

Blood Products and Insect Bites

Urticaria can be seen with blood transfusion. Bites or stings due to spiders, snakes, insects can produce urticaria by immunological as well as by non-immunological mechanism.

Contactants

Wide variety of contactants like drugs, dyes, cosmetics, tooth paste, fabrics, soaps etc. can be responsible for urticaria.

Drugs

Drugs can produce urticaria by immunological as well as by non-immunological mechanism. The common drugs are: penicillamine, sulfonamides, coedine, aspirin and other anti-inflammatory agents, insulin, morphine, thyroid and parathyroid extracts.

Endogenous Diseases

This includes lupus erythematosus, malignancies, polycythemia, psycological factors and endocrinal disorders.

Food

Food allergy usually results in acute or recurrent attacks of urticaria, starting within minutes or few hours of ingestion and lasting for few hours/days. Common foods are: nuts, fish, eggs, chocolate, tomato, milk, cheese etc. Preservatives and dyes in food are other important factors.

Genetic Diseases

It include heriditary angioedema and familial cold urticaria.

Physical Urticaria

It is a distinct group in which wheals occur in response to physical stimuli i.e. cold, heat, solar rays, pressure, vibrations and water. Dermographism is a type of physical urticaria in which firm stroking of skin causes an exaggeration of triple response (erythema, oedema, and flare).

Infections/Infestations

Urticaria has been seen with viral, bacterial, fungal and parasitic infections. Mechanism is believed to be immunological.

Treatment

It is essential to take very careful and detailed history and make a thorough physical examination to detect the cause. If cause is found, avoidance of that causative agent is obviously the treatment of choice. However, due to difficulty in identifying or eliminating such a factor, symptomatic treatment should be given. Antihistamine drugs (H_1 blocker) are the mainstay in the management of urticaria. The combination of H_1 and H_2 blocker (Cimetidine) may be effective in treatment of chronic urticaria. The tricyclic antidepressant (Doxipin) and β adrenergic agonist (Terbutaline) may be beneficial in a few cases. Systemic steroids are only indicated in very acute or recalcitrant cases.

ANGIO OEDEMA

This is a variant of urticaria in which subcutaneous tissue rather than dermis is mainly involved. It commonly affects the lips, periorbital tissues, genetalia and sometimes even tongue and larynx. Itching is usually absent.

Treatment is same as that of chronic urticaria. Acute cases require adrenaline and corticosteroids.

18

Drug Reactions

Adverse reactions to drugs are extremely common and are seen more often in the skin than in any other organ. Drug reaction may result from the drugs applied locally or administered systemically.

Mechanism of Drug Reactions

Drugs used in *Over Dosages* may produce toxicity or sometime there may be unwanted pharmacological action of the drug in usual dosages i.e. *Side Effect.* Administration of two or more drugs simultaneously after alters the effect of one or both drugs due to *Interaction* between drugs. The drug may produce any of the four classical types of *Allergic Reactions* i.e. type I to IV. It may produce different allergic reactions in the same individual at different times. Certain individuals may show an uncharacteristic response to drug i.e. *Idiosyncracy Ecological Imbalance* may be produced by certain drugs by altering the natural balance of micro-organism in G.I. tract. *Teratogenic and Other Foetal Defects* are well known due to certain drugs.

Types of Drug Reactions

Exanthematic Eruptions

This type of drug rash is the most common. The lesions are erythematous macules or maculopapules, which are usually distributed symmetrically and are commonly seen with ampicillin, gentamycin, phenylbutazone, gold, mercury and sulphonamides.

Urticaria

Urticaria can be produced either by a type I or type III allergic reaction. Some drugs act directly as histamine liberators. The drugs most commonly causing urticaria are: penicillin, aspirin, barbiturates, hydralazine, sulphonamides, coedine and morphine. Urticaria may accompany serum sickness reactions or systemic anaphylaxis.

Fixed Drug Eruptions

Fixed drug eruptions are circumscribed lesions that recur persistantly at the site with each administration of the allergenic drug. It is characterized by appearance of round or oval, dusky red patches that rapidly become raised, itchy and even bullous. Healing of the lesions leave behind a patch of hyperpigmentation. The common drugs responsible for fixed eruptions are: tetracyclines, sulphonamides, barbiturates, phenolpthalein and salicylates.

Lichenoid Drug Eruptions

The common drugs causing lichenoid eruptions are: heavymetals PAS, streptomycin, INH, tolbutamide, chlorpropamide and methyl dopa.

Exfoliative Dermatitis

The common drugs causing exfoliative dermatitis include gold, mercury, barbiturates, sulphonamides, phenylbutazone, PAS and hydantoin.

Acneiform Eruptions

Acneiform eruptions are commonly produced by ACTH, corticosteroids, androgens, INH, oral contraceptives, iodides and bromides.

Pigmentation

The common drugs responsible for pigmentation are: tetracycline, minocycline, chloroquine, mepacrine, heavy metals, clofazimine and chlorpromazine.

Bullous Eruptions

Bullous drug reaction can occur due to barbiturates, sulphonamides, meprobamate, nalidixic acid and nitrazepam. Pemphigus like eruption may be caused by penicillamine, betablockers and captopril.

Erythema Multiforme

The causative drugs include barbiturates, salicylates, sulphonamides, penicillin and hydantoin.

Eczematous Eruptions

These may be caused by methyldopa, sulphonamides, phenylbutazone and sulphonyl ureas.

Lupus Erythematosus like syndrome

can induce lupus erythematous like syndrome are: procainamide, hydralazine, INH and penicillamine.

Purpuric Eruptions

The causative drugs include arsenic, barbiturates, quinidine, sulphonamides, and meprobamate.

Erythema Nodosum

It is characterized by appearance of erythematous, painful and tender nodules, usually on the shins. The most common causes are streptococcal infection, tuberculosis, sarcoidosis, histoplasmosis and drugs (sulphonamides and oral contraceptives).

Alopecia

Alopecia may be induced by antimetabolites, anticoagulants, antithyroid and oral contraceptive drugs.

Photosensitivity

Drug reaction may be phototoxic or photoallergic. Various drugs causing photosensitivity are: psoralen, sulphonamides, griseofulvin, tetracycline, phenothiazine and thiazides.

Pityriasis Rosea Like Eruptions:

Drugs causing pityriasis rosea like eruptions are: gold. bismuth, barbiturates and captopril.

Toxic Epidermal Necrolysis

It is characterized by erythema, tenderness and extensive peeling off the skin leaving a raw surface like a scald. The common drugs responsible are: dephenhydantoin, phenylbutazone, chlorpropamide and sulphonamides.

Diagnosis

The diagnosis of drug reaction is based on detailed history and thorough clinical examination. Laboratory tests are almost valueless.

Diagnosis usually depends on the result of discontinuation of the drug and in some cases it may be possible to confirm it by giving a 'challenge' dose of the drug at a later date.

Treatment

The great majority of drug eruption subside within few days of stopping the drug. Milder cases require symptomatic treatment in the form of oral antihistamines and local application of soothing agents like calamine lotion. Severe reactions should be treated with systemic corticosteroids.

19

Lupus Erythematosus and Systemic Sclerosis

LUPUS ERYTHEMATOSUS (LE)

LE is a common collagen disorder of autoimmune aetiology which is generally divided into two types: Discoid lupus erythematosus and systemic lupus erythematosus.

Discoid Lupus Erythematosus (DLE)

DLE is a chronic scarring dermatosis of skin and mucous membrane. It chiefly affects the butterfly area of the face (cheeks, nose and central forehead), the scalp, the ears and occasionally the lips, the extremities and the trunk. Females are affected more often than males and average age of onset being 25-40 years.

Clinically, it is characterized by well defined, erythematous and scaly plaques with follicular plugging. The scales are large and adherent. When the scale is lifted, the keratin plugs can often be seen on its undersurface, giving a so called 'Carpet tack' appearance. The lesion spreads peripherally and tends to heal centrally by atrophy, scarring and pigmentary changes, usually depigmentation.

Lesions of mucous membrane are usually seen on the lower lips, where there is erythema, crusting, erosion and later scarring. On the scalp, the lesions produce cicatracial alopecia.

DLE may begin with single or multiple lesions and may become generalized. The lesions are usually precipitated or exacerbated by sunlight. The untreated lesions persist for years.

The diagnosis is confirmed by histopathological examination of biopsy of an active cutaneous lesion. Important histopathological

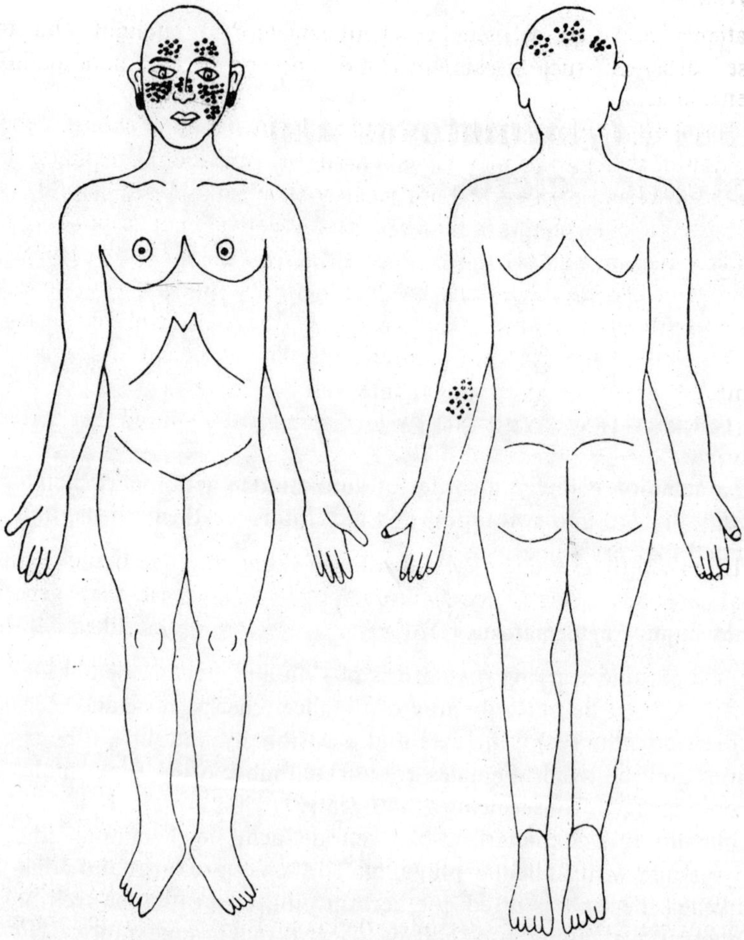

Fig. 19 Discoid lupus erythematosus:
Distribution of lesions

features are hyperkeratosis with follicular plugging, flattening of rete rigdges, hydropic degeneration of basal cell layer, periappendageal lymphocytic infiltration and dermal oedema. Immunofluorscence of involved skin reveals deposition of immunoglobulins (IgG, IgM and IgA) and complements in the basement membrane zone.

Treatment

Patients should be instructed to avoid exposure to sunlight and to use sun screens such as calamine lotion, zinc oxide and para-amino-benzoic acid.

Local application of corticosteroid is the treatment of choice. Penetration of the steroids may be enhanced by occlusion dressings. In resistant cases, intralesional corticosteroids injections are helpful.

Systemic chloroquine is required for the patients not responding to topical therapy and for those with extensive lesions. It is given in dosage of 200 mg twice daily for 3 to 4 weeks followed by once a day for about six months. The most serious side effect of this therapy is retinal damage. Hence, a careful ophthalmological examination should be performed at regular intervals.

Occasionally, systemic corticosteroids may be required for extensive and disseminated type of DLE.

Systemic Lupus Erythematosus (SLE)

SLE is a chronic multi-system disease of the connective tissue. Familial cases and a strong association of HLA B8 suggest that genetic factors play an part in the pathogenesis. Certain drugs like hydralazine, procainamide, hydantoin, INH and sulphonamide may precipitate SLE. It can occur at any age but usually seen in young adults with a marked female preponderance.

The cutaneous eruption consists of an illdefined, erythematous, slightly oedematous patch with fine scales, commonly affecting the malar region, nose and forehead but any other light exposed areas may be involved. The rash is usually precipitated or exacerbated by sunlight. DLE like lesions may occur in some cases. Occasionally, purpuric, urticarial, bullous, or erythema multiforme like lesions may be seen. Erythema and telangiectasia may occur on the nail folds, the thenar and the hypothenar eminences. The alopecia is a common feature and is usually diffuse and non-scarring. The oral mucous membrane if involved, shows superficial ulcers.

The systemic manifestations of SLE include fever, arthralgia or arthritis, nephrotic syndrome, pleurisy, pericarditis, hepato-splenomegaly, convulsion and psychic disturbances. Raynaud's phenomenon may be seen in some cases.

The clinical course tends to be quite variable with many exacerbations and remissions. If untreated, death occurs in a few years, usually from renal failure.

Laboratory Investigations

Laboratory findings include anaemia, leukopaenia, thrombocytopaea, raised ESR and a positive LE cell test in many cases. Presence of cellular casts and albumin in urine indicate renal damage. Demonstration of anti-nuclear antibodies (ANA) and antinative DNA antibodies (Anti-nDNA) in serum are the diagnostic test for SLE.

Histopathological changes in the skin lesion are almost similar to those found in lesion of DLE. Immunofluorescence of the involved and uninvolved skin shows deposition of immunoglobulins (IgG, IgM and IgA) and complements in the basement membrane zone.

Treatment

Precipitating and exacerbating factors (drugs, sun exposures) must be avoided. Systemic corticosteroid is the drug of choice and is to be given in the dosage of 30 to 80 mg per day. Once the disease appears to be under control, the dose should be tappered off as much as possible to a maintenance dose. Patients who do not respond well to corticosteroids may have to take immunosuppressive agents such as azathioprine or chlorambucil.

SYSTEMIC SCLEROSIS (SYSTEMIC SCLERODERMA)

Systemic sclerosis is an uncommon, multisystem disease of unknown aetiology. It is more often seen in females than in males, between the ages of 20 and 50. Raynaud's phenomenon is the most common presentation of systemic sclerosis which may precede other manifestations by months or even years. Cutaneous involvement usually starts peripherally on the hands and face but ultimately may involve the other parts of the body. The skin of the fingers, hands and face becomes tight and bound down to the underlying tissue. Facial changes consist of expression less facies, pinched nose, restricted mouth opening with radial furrows and thin lips. The fingers are smooth, shiny and taphered. Small painful gangrenous ulcers appear on the tips of the digits which can lead to progressive shortening of the affected digit. Pigmentary change may occur over forearm and chest in long standing cases. Intracutaneous and subcutaneous calcification occurs most commonly on the palmar aspects of terminal phalanges.

Systemic manifestations include oesophageal reflux, dysphagia, malabsorption, dyspnoea and uraemia.

The clinical course is variable but it is usually progressive and death may occur as a result of intercurrent infections or respiratory, cardiac or renal failure.

Laboratory Investigations

Antinuclear antibodies (ANA) is often present in very high titre. Other laboratory findings include anaemia, raised ESR and increased gammaglobulins. Barium swallow often shows dilatation and reduced mobility of the oesophagus. Skin biopsy is rarely helpful in doubtful cases. Immunofluorescence is negative.

Treatment

There is no satisfactory specific treatment. Patient should be advised to protect themselves from cold and trauma. Vasodilators, low molecular weight dextran, sympathectomy and stanozolol have been tried to alleviate the Raynaud's. D-penicillamine, systemic corticosteroids and immunosuppressive agents have all been tried with variable results. Symptomatic treatment for systemic involvement may be needed.

20

Genodermatoses

The term genodermatoses is restricted to those dermatological conditions which are genitically determined and may manifest at birth or later in life. They may be classified as dominant, recessive or sex linked depending on their mode of inheritance. The most common genodermatoses are:

ICHTHYOSIS

This is a group of inherited disorders, characterized by 'fish like' scales on the skin. There are two main forms: (a) ichthyosis vulgaris and (b) sex linked ichthyosis.

Ichthyosis Vulgaris

It is the most common form of ichthyosis which is transmitted by autosomal dominant genes. The peak age of onset is between 1 and 4 years. The skin shows small, white or light brown scales on the back and extensor surfaces of the extremities. Flexures of the limbs are usually spared. The disease is aggravated in winter season and improves during summer season. There is often an atopic history and keratosis pilaris. Accentuation of palmar and plantar creases may be present. The course of the disease is usually persistent and may worsen with age.

Treatment consists of topical application of emollients (vaseline, oil or lanoline) which helps in lubricating the skin and prevent excessive dryness. Keratolytic agents such as salicylic acid (2-5%), urea (5-10%), or retinoic acid (0.1%) are helpful. Systemic retinoids may be given only in severe cases.

Sex Linked Ichthyosis

This type of ichthyosis is inherited by a sex linked recessive gene and affects only males. It usually begins in early infancy and is characterized by large, dark, adherent scales on the front of the trunk, scalp, sides of face and extremities. The flexures may be moderately affected. The palms and soles are usually spared. Sex linked ichthyosis may be associated with corneal opacity. The course of the disease is persistent. Treatment is similar to that recommended for ichthyosis vulgaris.

NEUROFIBROMATOSIS (VON RECKLINGHAUSEN'S DISEASE)

Neurofibromatosis is a hereditary disease due to an autosomal dominant gene, affecting skin, nervous system, bones, mucous membranes and endocrine system.

Cutaneous findings include cafe-au-lait spots, freckling and multiple tumours. Cafe-au-lait spots are sharply defined, light brown oval patches, often 2-5 cm in length, commonly found on the trunk. Presence of freckle like spots in the axillae and perineum is a pathognomonic sign of the disease. The skin tumours are soft, skin coloured and sessile or pedunculated. They vary considerably in number and size. In some cases, tumours occurring in the course of peripheral nerves are felt as small, firm, discrete nodules. In rare instances, tumours may be grouped along the branches of a nerve to form a large irregular beaded mass (Plexiform neuroma).

Systemic manifestations of this syndrome may include mental retardation, epilepsy, spinal deformity, raised intracranial tension, acromegaly, hypertension and pricocious puberty.

There is no specific therapy except excision of troublesome tumours

EPILOIA (TUBEROUS SCLEROSIS)

Epiloia is inherited as an autosomal dominant gene. It is characterized by a classic triad of epilepsy, mental retardation and adenoma sebaceum. Adenoma sebaceum are small, discrete pink papules 1-5 mm, commonly found on the nasolabial folds, chin and cheeks. Other cutaneous manifestations of epiloia are the shagreen patch (connective tissue naevi), periungual fibromas, depigmented leaf shaped macules and cafe-au-lait spots. Systemic manifestations include mental retardation, epilepsy, ocular abnormalities (Phakomas) and renal hamartomas.

Adenoma sebaceum can be excised or removed by currettage and cautery or cryotherapy.

21

Skin Tumours

The tumours of the skin can be discussed under following heads:

Benign cutaneous tumours
Premalignant cutaneous tumours
Malignant cutaneous tumours

BENIGN CUTANEOUS TUMOURS

Seborrhoeic Keratoses

This is a common benign tumour of the epidermis occuring in elderly individuals. The lesions are sharply demarcated, dirty brown or black in colour, slightly raised with velvety or verrucous surface and often look as if they are 'stuck on' the surface of the skin. The size of the lesion varies from 1 mm to several centimeters. Occassionally, seborrhoeic keratosis may be pedunculated. The sites of predilection are the back, central chest, the face and the extremities. The sudden appearance and rapid increase in size and number of the lesions should arouse the suspicion of internal malignancy.

The most satisfactory treatment is currettage and electrodessication of the lesions. Chemical cautery and cryotherapy are also effective.

Keratoacanthoma

Keratoacanthoma is an uncommon benign tumour of the skin occurring in older individuals. This bears a striking resembalance both clinically and histopathologically to squamous cell carcinoma. The lesion consists of a firm, dome shaped, umblicated nodule usually single but may be multiple. The umblication is filled with a thick keratinous plug. The lesions occur mostly in sun exposed areas.

Many keratoacanthomas undergo spontaneous resolution with expulsion of keratinous plug and scar formation. The treatment is excision or currettage and cautery.

PREMALIGNANT CUTANEOUS TUMOURS

Solar Keratoses (Actinic Keratoses)

Solar keratoses are usually multiple, small, red, scaly maculopapular lesions in sun exposed areas of the skin. These lesions mainly occur in persons in or past middle life who have a repeated history of sun-exposure. It may evolve into squamous cell carcinoma. Solar keratosis are best treated by currettage and cauterization. Cryotherapy with liquid nitrogen also provides satisfactory results.

Bowen's Disease

It manifests as a persistent, slowly growing, red scaly plaque with sharp but irregular outline. The lesion in exposed areas are usually caused by exposure to sun and on unexposed skin by ingestion of arsenic. Lesions of Bowen's disease can occur on the glans penis (erythroplasia of Queyrat). Most effective treatment is currettage and electrodessication.

Other premalignant cutaneous tumours are arsenical keratoses, paget's disease and leukoplakia.

MALIGNANT CUTANEOUS TUMOURS

Basal Cell Carcinoma

Basal cell carcinoma is the commonest malignant tumour arising from the basal cell layer of the epidermis and chiefly affecting the upper central part of the face. It usually starts as a small, skin coloured papule which slowly enlarges peripherally and often undergoes central ulceration. This produces the classical picture of this 'rodent ulcer' with pearly rolled border. If basal cell carcinoma is left untreated for long periods of time, it eventually erode the underlying tissues. It rarely metastasizes. Basal cell carcinoma is occassionally present in other forms e.g. as brown pigmented lesions, sclerotic plaques, pedunculated nodules or flat red scaly macules with slightly elevated borders.

The factors that predispose a person to develop basal cell carcinoma are prolonged exposure to sunlight and rontgen rays, presence of burn scars and intake of arsenical salts.

Various effective treatment modalities are surgical excision, currettage and electrodessication, radiotherapy and cryotherapy. The choice of treatment depends on site and size of tumour and age of the patient.

Squamous Cell Carcinoma

Squamous cell carcinoma is a malignant metastatic tumour of epidermis which may arise as such or may complicate dermatosis like solar keratosis, leukoplakia, Bowen's disease, lupus vulgaris, chronic ulcers, scars etc. Clinically, squamous cell carcinoma of skin commonly presents as an indurated shallow ulcer with rolled out edges. Sometimes one may come across a verrucous and fungating lesion without ulceration. The regional lymphnodes may show enlargemant due to metastasis. Lesions may occur any where on the skin as well as on mucous membranes but the most commonly affected sites are the face, the dorsa of hands and forearm. the lower lip and the prepuce.

Squamous cell carcinoma is usually treated by surgical excision or radiotherapy. Very early lesions can be treated by currettage and electrodessication.

22

Sexually Transmitted Diseases

Sexually transmitted diseases are generally defined as those diseases that are transmitted principally by sexual contact. These can be classified as under due to:

1. Bacteria
   - Chancroid
   - Gonorrhoea
   - Donovanosis
   - Lymphogranuloma venereum.
2. Viruses
   - Condyloma acuminata
   - Herpes genitalis
   - Molluscum contagiosum
   - Acquired immuno deficiency syndrome (AIDS)
3. Spirochaete
   - Syphilis
4. Fungi
   - Candidiasis
5. Parasites
   - Scabies
   - Pediculosis
6. Protozoan
   - Trichomoniasis

SYPHILIS

It is a chronic, infectious and contagious disease caused by Treponema pallidum. The infection is capable of affecting all the organs and systems of the body but the skin, the mucous membranes, the eye, the central nervous system and cardiovascular system are mainly involved.

The disease is often transmitted by sexual contact, rarely by kissing, through transfusion of infected blood and by indirect contact with infected objects. It may also be transmitted from infected mother to child during intrauterine period.

Classification

The two main types of syphilis are:

Acquired and Congenital

Acquired syphilis can be classified as follows:

(a) Early infectious phase endures less than two years and includes:

Primary syphilis,

Secondary syphilis, and

Early latent syphilis

(b) Late non infectious phase is of more than two year's duration and includes:

Late latent syphilis,

Tertiary syphilis,

Cardiovascular and neurosyphilis

Congenitial syphilis can be subdivided into early, late and stigmata stage.

Primary Syphilis

Clinical Features

The incubation period is 10-90 days. The primary lesion is often found on the sites subject to trauma during intercourse. It begins as a small red papule which rapidly becomes eroded giving rise to an ulcer. The ulcer is called ihe 'primary chancre' and has a well defined margin, indurated base with a clean granulation tissue in the floor.

It exudes clear serum on manipulation. The primary chancre is usually single, painless and indolent. The inguinal lymphadenopathy develops usually within one week of the onset of the chancre. The lymph nodes are multiple, discrete, non tender and rubbery in consistency, Involvement is often bilateral. The primary chancre tends to heal without treatment in 3-10 weeks leaving behind a thin atrophic scar.

Common sites in men are the corona sulcus, glans, meatus, prepuce, frenum and shaft of penis. and in women, the labia majora and minora, cervix, clitoris and fourchette. In homosexual men, the chancre may be seen at or near the anus. Extragenital chancres may be seen on the lips, the fingers, the tongue, the eyelids and the nipples.

Secondary Syphilis

The average interval between the appearance of primary chancre and the onset of the secondary lesions is from 6 to 8 weeks. Various manifestations of secondary syphilis are:

(a) *Prodromal Phase*

It consists of malaise, low grade fever, loss of weight and headache.

(b) *Skin Rashes*

These may be macular, papular, papulo-squamous or pustular. The lesions are dull red in colour, round or oval in shape, non pruritic and distributed bilaterally symmetrically on the flexures. The papular lesions in warm, moist regions of the body such as perianal region, become large and hypertrophic with broad base and flat top and are called 'condylomata lata'. Skin lesions heal slowly leaving hypo or hyperpigmented areas.

(c) *Mucous Membrane Lesions*

The typical lesions of mucous membranes are mucous patches, which are slightly raised, grey white in colour and have a tendency to ulcerate. These patches may coalesce to form 'snail tract ulcers'. The common sites are the mucosa of the mouth, genital, pharynx and larynx.

(d) *Lypmphadenopathy*

Lymph nodes of suboccipital, cervical, axillary, epicondylar and inguinal regions are usually enlarged, discrete, nontender and rubbery in consistency.

(e) *Systemic Manifestations*

The rare manifestations include hepatospleenomegaly, anterior uveitis and nephrotic syndrome.

Condyloma lata and mucous patches are highly infectious lesions. The lesions tend to heal without treatment in 2-3 months. Occasionally, there is recurrence of secondary lesions within the first 2 years of infection.

Early Latent Syphilis

When the symptoms and signs of secondary syphilis disappear, the disease is said to latent and may persist upto end of the second year of the infection. The patient with latient syphilis has no clinical signs and symptoms of the disease and diagnosis depends on positive serological tests. Cereberospinal fluid examination is normal in early latent syphilis.

Late Latent Syphilis

After the second year of the infection, the disease enters the late latent phase. This stage is asymptomatic, non contagious and may last for months, years or for the rest of the patient's life. Diagnosis is made by history and positive serological tests.

Cerebrospinal fluid should be examined to exclude asymptomatic neurosyphilis.

Tertiary Syphilis

The most typical lesion of tertiary syphilis is gumma, which may appear between 3 and 10 years after the primary lesion. Gumma usually occur in skin, mucous membrane, subcutaneous tissue, bones or visceras. Cutaneous gummas are nodular, squamous or subcutaneous type. These tends to heal at the centre leaving thin, atrophic 'tissue paper' scar. Mucosal gummas are painless, localized swellings which break down to form characteristic 'punched out' ulcers.

Bony gummas are usually seen in tibia and cranial bones, resulting in osteitis and osteomyelitis. Gummas of visceras are very rare.

Cardiovascular and Neurosyphilis

These are very rare and occur in about 10% of untreated syphilitics.

The manifestations of cardiovascular syphilis include uncomplicated aortitis, aortic regurgitation, angina pectoris, and aortic aneurism.

In neurosyphilis, various combination of meningeal, vascular and parenchymatous involvent may occur. Meningovascular syphilis produces signs and symptoms identical to those of meningitis of other causes. Parenchymatous neurosyphilis includes tabes dorsalis (affecting the spinal cord) and general paralysis of insane (affecting the brain).

Diagnosis

Diagnosis is made by a combination of clinical examination, dark ground examination and serological tests.

1. Dark ground examination of serous exudates from ulcer or from moist secondary lesions may reveal treponema pallidum. T. pallidum is a delicate, corkscrew-like spirochaete with characteristic movements which include rotation and forward movements, coil compression and expansion and undulation and angulation.
2. Serological tests for syphilis are divided into non-specific and specific tests. Nonspecific tests include cardiolipin wasserman reaction (WR) and venereal disease research laboratory (VDRL) test. These become positive about two weeks after the appearance of the primary chancre.

   Specific tests include treponema immobilization (TPI) test, absorbed fluorescent treponemal antibody (FTA-ABS) test, treponema pallidum haemagglutination (TPHA) test and Reiter protein complement fixation (RPCF) test.

FTA-ABS test is generally the first to become positive in early syphilis. After adequate treatment of early syphilis, non specific tests become negative within 3-6 months in majority of the cases.

Treatment

Treatment of Early Infectious Stage

(a) Benzathine penicillin G, 2.4 million units intramuscularly at a single session (1.2 million in each buttock);

or

(b) Aqueous procain penicillin G, 600,000 units intramuscularly for 8-10 days.

Treatment of Late Non-Infectious Stage

1. Benzathine penicilin G, 3 million units intramuscularly, weekly for 3 weeks;

or

2. Aqueous procain penicillin G, 600,000 units intramuscularly, daily for 15-20 days.

Patients allergic to penicillin should receive erythromycin or tetracyline in the dosage of 500 mg six hourly for 15 days in early syphilis, and 30 days in late syphilis or in latent syphilis of more than a year's duration.

Congenital Syphilis

Congenital syphilis results from the transmission of mother's syphilis to the fetus. This usually occurs in about the 19th week of pregnancy when T. pallidum passes through the placenta into the foetal circulation. Congenital syphilis is divided into early, late and stigmata.

1. Early Congential Syphilis: It usually develops before the age of two and changes noted are basically these of secondary syphilis. Skin lesions may be vesicobullous, macular, papular or papulosquamous. The palms, soles, buttocks and genitalia are frequently affected.

Mucous patches occur in the oral mucosa and nose. In nose, it causes syphilitic rhinitis leading on to obstruction along with osteitis and may lead to collapse of the bridge of the nose, resulting in 'saddle nose'. Perioral lesions cause radiating fissures. Other mani festations include osteochondritis of long bones, hepatospleenome galy, lymph adenitis and iritis.

2. Late Congenital Syphilis: It is seen after two years of age. Various manifestations are eight nerve deafness, bilateral hydrarthrosis of the knee joints (Clutton's joint), interstitial keratitis, perforation of palate, destruction of nasal septum, periostitis of tibia (sabre tibia), bony massses of skull (Parrot's nodes) and frontal bossing.

3. The Stigmata: The stigmata are sequellae of lesions of congenital syphilis. These include saddle nose, Hutchinson's teeth (pegged shaped), Rhagdes (scar at the angle of mouth), corneal opacities, gummatous scars, optic atrophy and deafness.

Diagnosis

In early congenital syphilis, dark ground examination of serum from moist lesions of skin and mucous membranes will show T. pallidum.

Serological tests are reactive but it is essential to exclude the passive transfer of reagins from the mother (which disappear within 6 months).

Treatment

For early congential syphilis: Benzathin penicillln G, 50,000 units/kg of body weigh at a single session; or Procain penicillin, 500,000 units/kg of body weight, to be given in divided dosage for 10 days. In late congenital syphilis, the scheme of treatment is similar with the total dosage again based on body weight. Patient, over 12 years of age, require same doses as for adult late syphilis.

CHANCROID

It is an acute, infectious, autoinocular infection of the genitalia, caused by Haemophilus ducreii.

Clinical Features

Incubation period is short usually 1-5 days, rarely longer. Lesions are small, red painful papules or pustules which rapidly break down to form sharply circumscribed ulcers with undermined edges. The base is formed by vascular granulation tissue and often covered with grey purulent exudates. Lesions are tender to touch and bleed easily on manipulation. They are usually multiple as a result of autoinoccu-lation. Ulcers are not indurated hence the term 'soft chancre' is some-times used to describe chancroid.

Common location of ulcers in men are the mucousal surface of pre-puce or frenum of prepuce, and in women, the labia, clitoris, four-chaette and vestibule. The inguinal lymph glands, usually of one side, become painful and enlarged within a week of appearance of soft chancre. The nodes are metted together to form a inflammatory bubo which may suppurate and rupture to form a large ulcer in the groin.

Phagedenic ulceration, phimosis, uretheral fistulae and uretheral stricture are the other complications of the disease.

Diagnosis

In each case, dark field examination should be performed to rule out syphilis.

(1) Make a smear from the ulcers or from the pus as aspirated from unruptured bubo and stain with gram's stain or wright's stain. H. ducreii are short, gram negative bacilli and are usually arranged in chains giving the appearance of a 'School of fish'.

(2) Culture of the smear or pus can be done on special media containing fresh blood.

(3) Biopsy of lesions will show superficial necrosis, pallisading and endothelial proliferation of blood vessels, degenertion of vessel wall and occasionally thrombosis, and infiltration by plasma cells and lymphocytes in the deeper zone.

Treatment

1. Sulphadiazine, 2 gm orally at once, then 1 gm every 6 hourly for 10-15 days; or
2. Co-trimoxazole, or two tablets twice a day for 7-10 days; or
3. Streptomycin, 1 gm intramuscularly daily for 7-14 days; or
4. Tetracycline, 500 mg orally, 6 hourly for 10-20 days.

If bubo is present, the combined treatment with streptomycin and sulphonamide is effective and fluctuating bubo should be aspirated, never incised.

GRANULOMA INGUINALE (DONOVANOSIS)

This is an uncommon, chronic granulomatous infection involving the genitals, perineum and groins. It is caused by an organism called Donovania granulomatis.

Clinical Features

Incubation period is uncertain but appear to vary from 7 days to 30 days in majority of the cases. The lesions start as painless red papules which progress to form beefy red granulomatous ulcers with characteristic rolled edges. The lesions may spread widely and involve the adjacent areas by autoinocculation. There is little or no tendency to spontaneous healing. Subcutaneous granulomas may develop in the inguinal region and are called 'pseudobuboes'. They may breakdown producing granulomatous ulcers. There may be secondary infection, especially with vincent's organism producing phagedenic ulcerations with tissue destruction. Chronic and long standing cases may show carcinomatous changes.

Diagnosis

Diagnosis is based on demonstration of donovan bodies in the mononcuclear cells in the tissue smears or in the biopsy taken from an ulcer. Donovan bodies are gram negative curved bacilli and are usually recognised by their characteristic, bipolar staining ('Safety pin' appearance). Culture of organisms require special media i.e. yolk sac of chicken eggs.

Treatment

1. Streptomycin, 1 gm, twice a day for 10-20 days; or
2. Tetracycline, 500 mg 6 hourly, orally for 10-20 day; or
3. Cotrimoxazole, two tablets twice daily for 10-20 days.

LYMPHOGRANULOMA VENEREUM (LGV)

This is an uncommon, sexually transmitted disease caused by chlamydia trachomatis.

Clinical Features

The incubation period appears to be variable but is usually between 1 to 4 weeks. The primary genital lesion is usually a single, small vesicle or papule which may ulcerate. The lesion is asymptomatic and transient, often unnoticed. In men, the primary lesion usually appears on the glans penis, the coronal sulcus, the prepuce or the shaft of the penis.

Unilateral or bilateral inguinal lymphadenitis usually appears a few days to a few weeks after the primary lesion. The lymph nodes are enlarged, tender and metted together. The skin over the metted nodes may have a dusky red discolouration. The enlarged nodes are present below and above the inguinal ligament (the groove sign). Femoral and iliac nodes may be involved. Suppuration of nodes leads to formation of multiple abscesses which rupture to produce multiple sinuses. Mild constitutional symptoms may be present.

Late and chronic manifestations of LGV are scarring in the inguinal region, genital elephantiasis and ano-rectal syndrome. Genital elephantiasis is due to lymphodema caused by distruction and distortion of lymphatic drainage. Ano-rectal syndrome consists of proctitis, rectal strictures, rectal fistulae and perirectal abscesses. It is more commonly seen in females.

Diagnosis

The diagnosis of LGV is usually made on the basis of a characteristic clinical picture, culture of C. trachomatis, intradermal tests, complement fixation tests or microimmune fluorescent tests.

Treatment

1. Tetracyline, 500 mg 6 hourly, orally for 2-3 weeks; or
2. Sulphonamide, 1 gm 6 hourly, orally for 2-3 weeks; or
3. Cotrimoxazole, two tablets twice a day for 2-3 weeks; or
4. Erythromycin, 500 mg 6 hourly orally for 2-3 weeks.

Fluctuant abscesses should be aspirated, but should never be excised.

GONORRHEA

It is a common, acute, infectious disease involving the genitourinary tract of both sexes, caused by Neisseria gonorrhoeae.

Clinical Features

The incubation period is usually 2-5 days. Male presents with burning or discomfort on micturition followed by a purulent uretheral discharge. Females are usually asymptomatic or may present with dysurea and vaginal discharge. Prepubertal girls present with purulent vaginal discharge and redness and swelling of vulva.

Oropharyngeal gonorrhoea may result from oral coitus and is characterized by pharyngitis or tonsillitis. Anorectal gonorrhoea may result from anal coitus in passive homosexuals and is chacterized by rectal discharge and tenesmus. Gonococcal conjunctivitis is seen in neonates and is characterized by conjunctivitis and purulent discharge. In men, the complications of gonorrhoea are tysonitis, litteritis, epididymo-orchitis, stricture urethera, periuretheral abscess, conjunctivitis and arthritis. In women, the complications are skenitis, bartholinitis, salphingitis and pelvic inflammation.

Diagnosis

A definite diagnosis of gonorrhoea depends upon identificatification of gonococci by gram's staining and/or culture. To prepare a stained slide, the secretion from the site of the infection is spread evenly and thinly on the surface of the glass slide and stained with gram's staining. The positive smear shows gram negative, reniform diplococci within the polymorphonuclear leukocytes.

Gonococci can be cultured on modified Thyer martin medium. The colonies of N. gonorrhoea ferments only glucose.

Direct and indirect immunofluorescent techniques may be used in the diagnosis of gonorrhoea.

Treatment

1. Aqueous procain penicillin G, 4.8 million units, intramuscularly single dose together with 1 gm of probenecid orally; or
2. Ampicillin, 3.5 gm orally with 1 gm probenecid; or
3. Cotrimoxazole, 4 Tab. twice a day for 2-4 days; or
4. Norfloxacine, 800 mg orally as a single dose; or
5. Spectinomycin hydrochloride, 2 gm intramuscularly, single injection.

The last two drugs are also effective in penicillin resistant Gonococcal infection.

Acquired Immunodeficiency Syndrome (AIDS)

The acquired immunodeficiency syndrome has emerged as one of the most gruesome and dreadful disease of human beings. It was first described in U.S.A. in 1981 as a severe unexplained immunodeficiency.

Pathogenesis

This condition is caused by human immunodeficiency virus (HIV). This is of 2 types: HIV-1 and HIV-2. This virus belongs to the family Retroviridae. A special protein on the surface of HIV allows the virus to attach itself and penetrate into helper T_4 lymphocytes which are the master cells in body's immune defence mechanism. When the virus enters a T_4 lymphocyte, RNA based retrovirus uses its enzyme, reverse—transcriptase, to translate its genetic information into DNA which integrates into host cell DNA. The integrated viral genome now takes over complete control of the host cell to replicate its own genes thus converting infected T_4 lymphocytes into virus factories. The viruses emerge from the infected cell and then infect fresh T_4 lymphocytes. HIV has a specific tropism for T_4 lymphocytes. The basis of this selective tropism lies in the fact that T_4 cells appear to possess a surface receptor for this virus.

Mode of Spread

Disease is acquired by penetrative sexual intercourse (hetrosexual or homosexual), deep kissing, contact with blood, blood products, donated semen or body tissues/organs.

The most majority of contact with HIV infected blood involves transfusion of unscreened blood or the use of unsterilized syringes and needles. Mother to child transfer occurs in utero and during or shortly after birth. This disease occurs mainly in homosexuals, intravenous drug abusers, haemophiliacs etc.

Clinical Features

Clinically patient develops fever, rash, lymphoadenopathy, fatigue, night sweats, persistent diarrhoea, malignancies like Kaposi sarcoma and lymphoma limited to the brain and frequent infections with opportunistic pathogens. They include:

1. Parasitic infections: Pneumocystis carinii, toxoplasmosis, cryptosporidiosis and strongyloidosis
2. Fungal infections: Candidosis and cryptococcosis
3. Bacterial infections: Atypical mycobacteriosis
4. Viral infections: Cytomegalovirus, Herpesvirus type 1 and 2 an[illegible] progressive multifocal leucoencephalopathy presumed to be [illegible]ed by Papovavirus.

Laboratory Diagnosis

A. *Indirect Tests*

1. Lymphopaenia (below 2000/cu mm): This is because of the involvement of T_4 lymphocytes. There is persistent reduction of T_4 (helper) lymphocytes. T_8 (cytotoxic) lymphocytes are normal or increased. Therefore $T_4 : T_8$ ratio is decreased (normal 60: 30=2, in AIDS 15 : 30=1/2).
2. Other indirect tests include: cutaneous anergy, poor lymphocyte responsiveness to mitogens and antigens, reduced cytotoxicity, defective interferon production and circulatory immune complexs.

B. *Specific Tests*

These include detection of anti-HIV antibodies by enzyme-linked immunosorbent assay test, characterization of antigenic fractions by Western-blot technique, detection of HIV in infected cells by immunofluorescence and isolation of HIV in T_4 cell lines.

Remarkable progress has been made towards treatment of HIV infection. Various drugs like azidothymidine, cyclosporin and HPA-23 have been tried with variable results.

PLATE IX

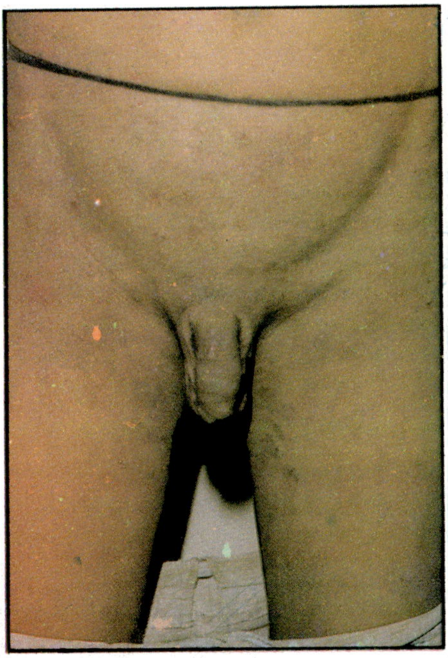

SCABIES

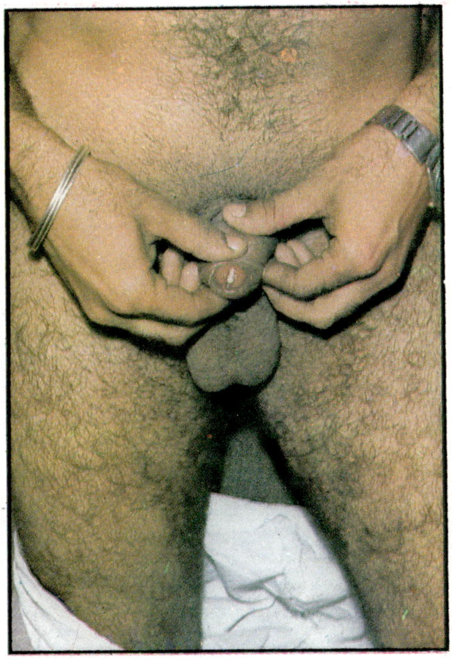

GONORRHEA

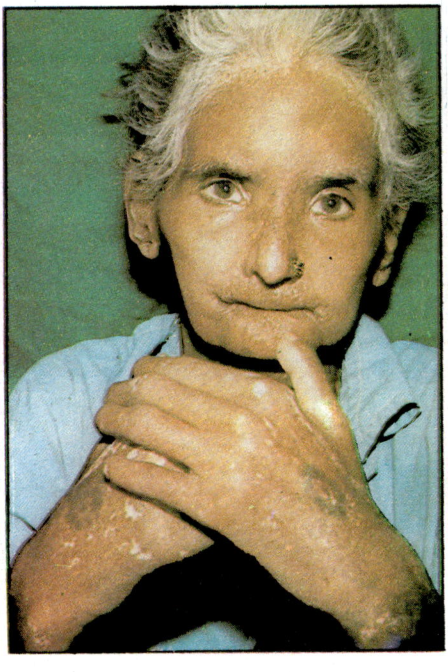

SYSTEMIC SCLEROSIS

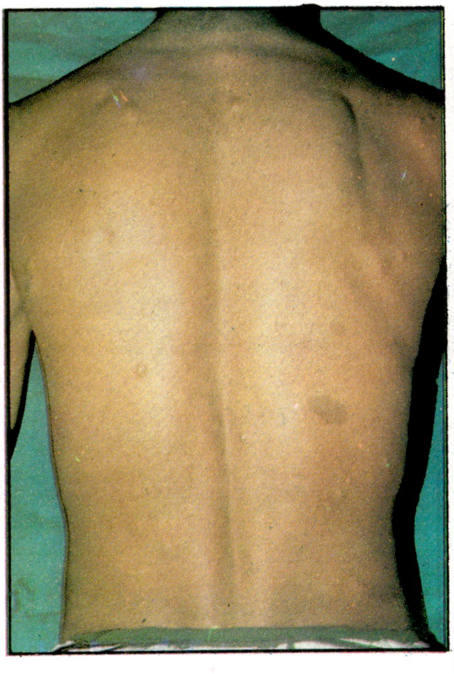

NEUROFIBROMATOSIS

PLATE X

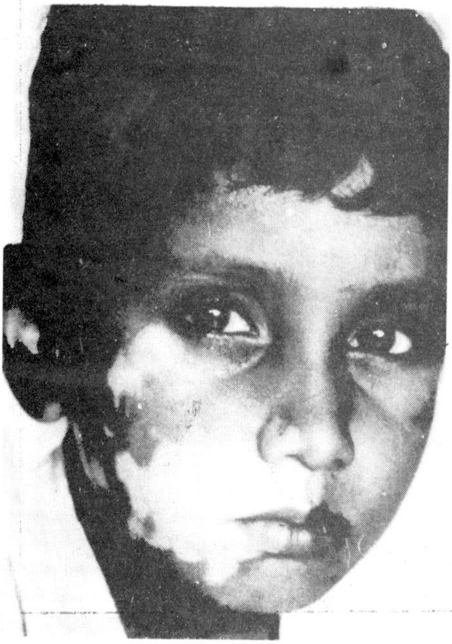

VITILIGO

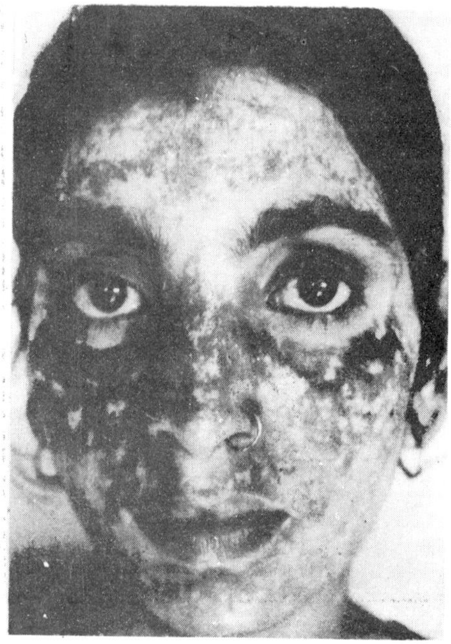

MELASMA

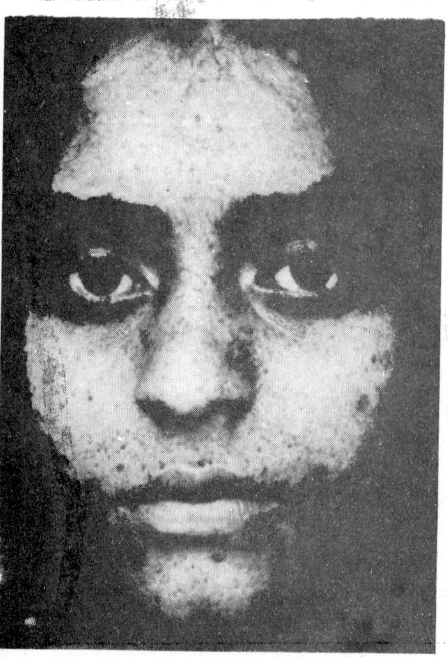

FRECKLES

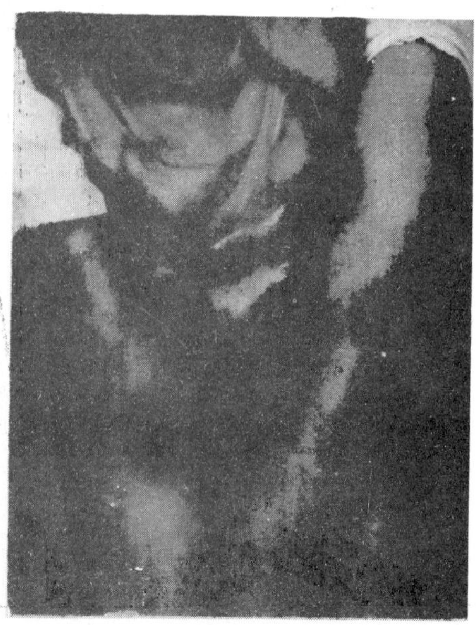

FIXED DRUG ERUPTION

PLATE XI

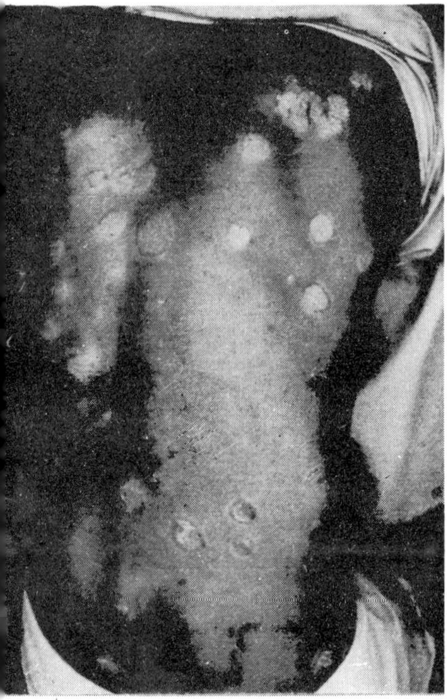

PSORIASIS

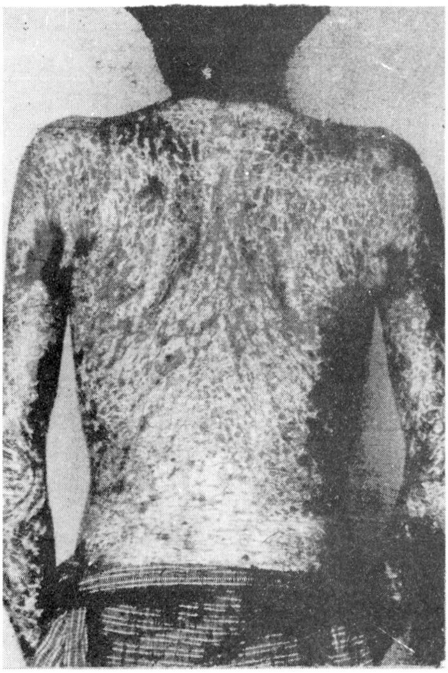

PSORIATIC ERYTHRODERMA

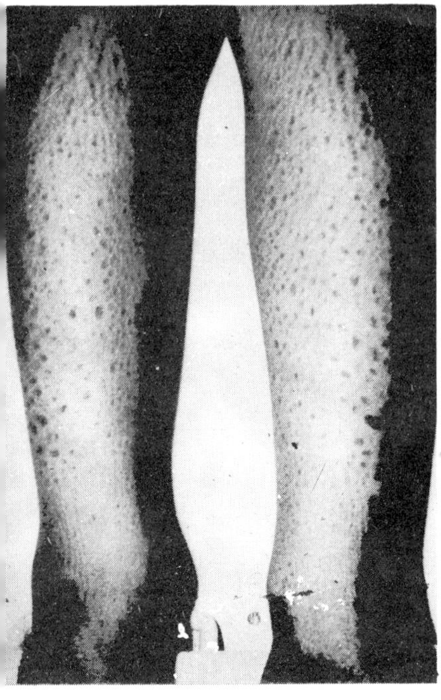

ICHTHYOSIS

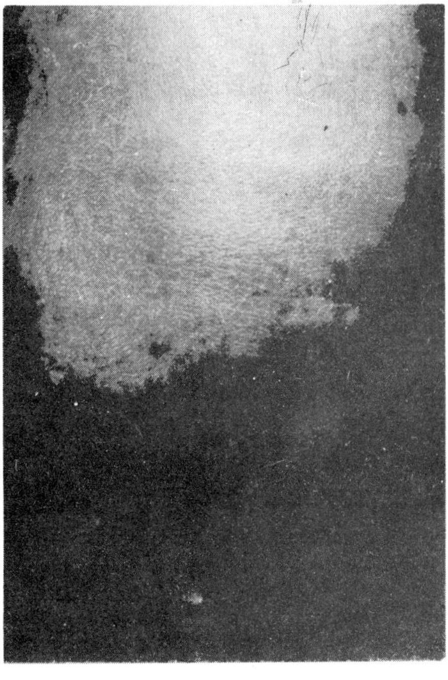

ALOPECIA UNIVERSALIS

PLATE XII

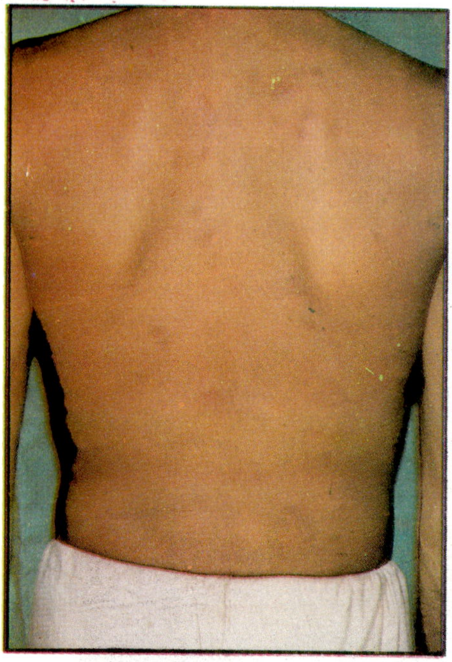

SECONDARY SYPHILIS

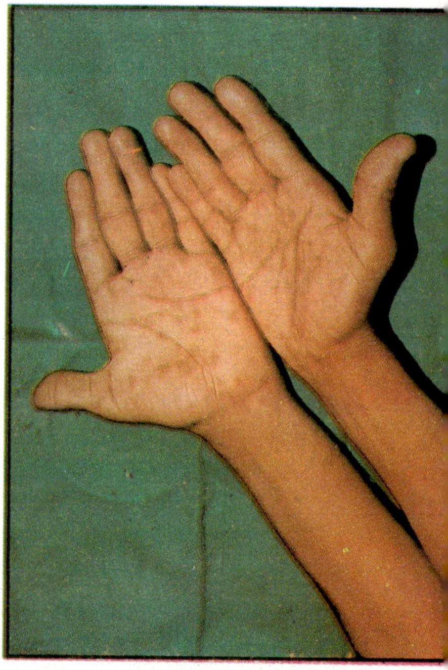

SECONDARY SYPHILIS

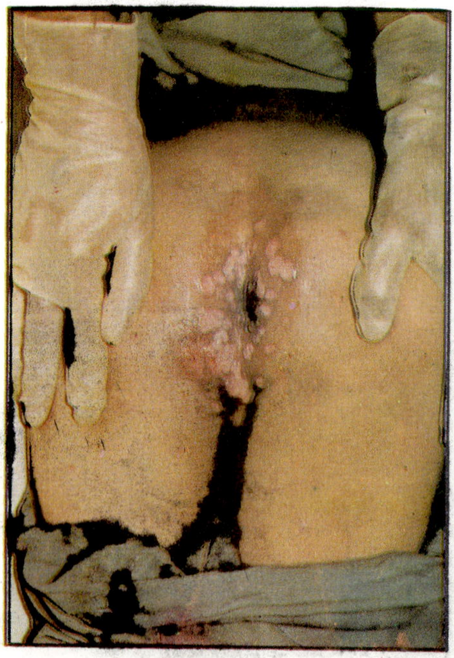

CONDYLOMA LATA

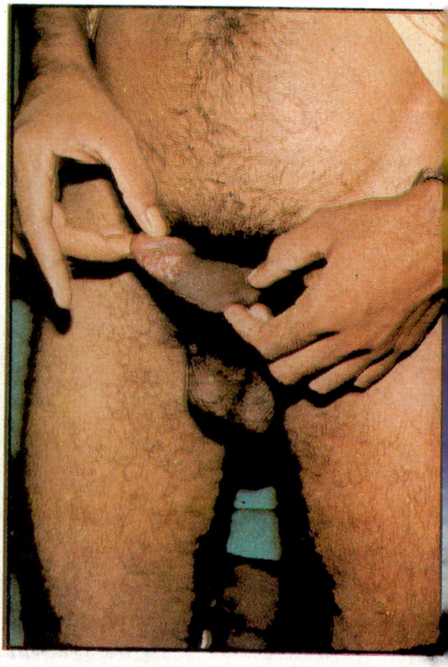

CHANCROID

23

Leprosy

Leprosy is often defined as a chronic disease resulting from infection with Mycobacterium leprae affecting primarily peripheral nerves and secondarily involve skin and certain other tissues.

Epidemiology

Two factors are required for the spread of leprosy, a susceptible individual and contact with M. leprae. Exact mechanism of transmission is not clear. Three possible routes of transmission are: the respiratory tract, the gastro-intestinal tract and the skin. Other factors which can affect transmission are: insect bite, over crowding and severe malnutrition. Age confers no exemption from leprosy infection. Children and young adults are more susceptible to infection.

Pathogenesis and Classification of Leprosy

The great majority of people have a complete resistance to infection with M. leprae and hence no disease develops in them. Only a proportion of infected persons develop signs of the disease after the usual incubation period of 2-5 years. The signs of the disease vary according to the degree of specific resistance of the host. Those with fairly high resistance develop tuberculoid leprosy, while those with poor or no resistance get lepromatous leprosy. Between these two extremes, there is wide range or spectrum of variations in resistance which are reflected in borderline group of leprosy.

The classification of leprosy is based on the clinical, bacteriological, immunological and histological findings. There are two stable polar types: Lepromatous (LL) and tuberculoid (TT) and two unstable types: indeterminate (I) and borderline (B). The borderline type has been subdivided into borderline tuberculoid (BT), mid borderline (BB) and borderline lepromatous (BL), according to their position with reference to the polar types.

Clinical Features

The clinical manifestations of leprosy are numerous and varied which are more often the result of host response to the presence of bacilli.

Indeterminate Leprosy (I)

Indeterminate leprosy appears as one or few hypopigmented or erythematous macules, one or a few cm in diameter. Margins of the lesions vary from ill defined to well defined. The lesions are distributed in asymmetrical pattern, often on the face and the trunk. Some sensory loss may be demonstrable but it is usually absent. The peripheral nerves usually remain normal. Indeterminate leprosy may heal spontaneously or may develop into tuberculoid, lepromatous or borderline leprosy. Bacteriologically, skin smears are often negative but occasionally a few bacilli can be demonstrated. Histologically, it is characterized by non-specific inflammatory reaction. Rarely, acid fast bacilli may be seen in dermal nerve fibrils. Immunologically, the lepromin test is usually positive, but may be negative in some cases.

Tuberculoid Leprosy (TT)

Clinically, it is characterized by presence of single or few, sharply defined, hypopigmented or erythematous macules or plaques. The surface is dry, hairless and anaesthetic. A thickened nerve trunk may be palpable in the vicinity of the lesion. Bacteriologically, the skin smears do not show any bacilli. Histologically, it is characterized by the presence of epitheloid cell granuloma with large number of lymphocytes eroding into the basal layer of the epidermis. Dermal nerves are heavily infilterated and may be completely destroyed. Acid fast bacilli are invariably absent. Immunologically, the lepromin test is strongly positive.

Borderline Tuberculoid Leprosy (BT)

Clinically, the skin lesions resemble those of tuberculoid type, but they are less sharply defined and are too numerous for TT. Often satellite lesions lie near the edges of larger lesions. Dryness, scaling, hairloss and loss of sensations tend to be less pronounced than in

TT. Several of the large peripheral nerves are being affected asymmetrically. Bacteriologically, the skin smears show slight positivity. Histologically, it is characterized by presence of epetheliod cell granuloma with foreign body giant cells and moderate amount of lymphocytes in the superficial dermis. There is narrow clear subepidermal zone. Dermal nerves are moderately swollen by cellular infiltrate and few acid fast bacilli may be demonstrated within dermal nerves. Immunologically, the lepromin test is positive.

Mid borderline Leprosy (BB)

Clinically, the skin lesions may be macules, plaques, annular, punched out, bizarre or nodules or a combination of any or all of these in a single patient, distributed asymmetrically. There will usually be many skin lesions, though not as numerous as in LL. The edges may be well defined in one area and poorly demonstrated elsewhere. Punched out lesion is characteristic of midborderline leprosy which has an ill defined sloping outer margin and a punched out central portion. Sensory impairment in the lesions is minimal. Nerve damage is variable. Bacteriologically, the skin smears are usually positive for acid fast bacilli. Histologically, there is an epitheloid cell granuloma with scanty lymphocytes and no giant cells. There is clear subepidermal zone. Dermal nerves show slight swelling and cellular infiltrate. Acid fast bacilli are present in moderate number. Immunologically, the lepromin test is usually negative.

Borderline Lepromatous (BL)

Clinically, it is characterized by presence of multiple papules, nodules or plaques. The surface of the lesion is usually smooth and shiny with ill defined edges. The lesions tend to be disposed in roughly symmetrical fashion. Some of lesions may resemble those of BB. There is little or no sensory loss. Several nerves are likely to be involved. Bacteriologically, the skin smears are positive. Histologically, there is macrophage granuloma with heavy infiltrate of lymphocytes. Dermal nerves show peculiar laminated appearance. A large number of acid fast bacilli are present. Immunologically, the lepromin test is negative.

Lepromatous Leprosy (LL)

Clinically, it is characterized by presence of multiple macules, papules or nodules, distributed bilaterally symmeterically. Sometimes diffuse cutaneous infiltration may be seen. The lesions are hypopigmented or erythematous, round or oval in shape with ill defined borders and a smooth and shiny surface. There is no sensory loss. Peripheral nerve involvement occurs later in the disease, which is bilateral and symmetrical resulting in 'glove and stocking' type of anaesthesia. Early nodules are commonly found on the face, especially the ears, but any part of the body may be affected. There is loss of eye brows and eye lashes (Madrosis). Diffuse infiltration and nodular lesions of the face may result in a change called 'Leonine facies'. Invasion of nasal mucosa may cause nasal stuffiness, epistaxis, perforation and collapse of nose (Saddle nose deformity). Other manifestations include iritis, keratitis, gynaecomastia, lymphadenopathy, atrophy of the muscles of the hands and feet, shortening of digits and trophic ulceration. Bacteriologically, smears are always highly positive for acid fast bacilli. Histologically, there is diffuse infiltration with vacoulated, foamy macrophages laden with acid fast bacilli. Lymphocytes, if present, are usually scanty. The epidermis is flattened and is separated from dermis by a clear subepidermal zone. Immunologically, the lepromin test is always negative.

Diagnosis of Leprosy

Diagnosis of leprosy can be made if one or more of the following cardinal signs of the disease are present. These are: (1) loss of sensation, (2) enlargement of peripheral nerves in specific sites and (3) demonstration of acid fast bacilli (AFB) in a skin smear.

Loss of Sensation

Loss of sensation to touch, pain and temperature of individual skin lesions or in the distribution of a large peripheral nerve is tested by means of a wisp of cotton wool, a pin and with cold and hot test tube.

Enlargement of Peripheral Nerves

Certain peripheral nerves must be routinely examined in every suspected leprosy patient. These are: the great auricular nerve, the ulnar, the median, the radial, the common peroneal and the posterior tibial.

Demonstration of Acid Fast Bacilli

The diagnosis of leprosy is confirmed by demonstration of AFB by slit skin smear method. Material for the smear is obtained from the suspected lesion as well as from the sites commonly affected in lepromatous leprosy usually the forehead, ear lobes and chin. The skin is cleaned and pinched up between thumb and forefinger. A small but deep incision is made with a sharp scalpel. The blade is scrapped several times and the material thus obtained is smeared onto a glass slide. The smear is stained with Zeihl Neelson's stain and examined under oil immersion lens. The bacilli are seen as red rods which may be solid staining (living) or fragmented or beaded (non living). The density of living and non living bacilli in a smear is known as bacteriological index (BI). The morphological index (MI) indicates the percentage of living bacilli and is useful index for determining the infectiousness of the patient.

Lepra Reactions

Sudden and acute bouts of exacerbation seen during the course of the disease, even during treatment, are termed as 'reactions'. These reactions are classified into type I and type II (erythema nodosum leprosum-ENL).

Type I: *Reaction*

It is due to rapid change in cell mediated immunity either for better or worse. It commonly occurs in patients with borderline disease (BL, BB, BT), whose immunological status is unstable. Under treatment, there may be a shift towards tuberculoid pole of spectrum, a 'upgrading reaction'. In untreated patients, the shift may be towards the lepromatous pole of the spectrum, a 'downgrading reaction'. Reaction in either case consists of erythema and swelling of some or all the existing skin lesions. One or more peripheral nerves become swollen and tender and motor disturbances may lead to permanent paralysis.

Type 2: *Reaction* (*Erythema Nodosum Leprosum-ENL*)

It is due to antigen antibody reaction with the formation of immune complexes which are deposited in various tissues. It occurs most commonly in LL and rarely in BL. Type 2 reaction may be triggered by several factors: Ingestion of antileprosy drugs, physical and mental stress, intercurrent infection, pregnancy and injuries.

Clinically, the skin lesions are tender, red nodules or plaques, distributed bilaterally and symmetrically mainly on the face, arms and thighs. The lesions appear in crops and disappear spontaneously within 2-3 days leaving behind a bluish grey discolouration. In severe cases, there may be central necrosis, pustulation, and even ulcers. Systemic manifestations of reaction are fever, malaise, joint pain, swollen and tender nerves. epistaxis, iridocyclitis, lymphadenitis and orchitis.

Treatment of Leprosy

Drugs available for the treatment of leprosy are: dapsone, rifampicine, clofazimine, ethionamide, prothionamide and thiacetazone.

Dapsone (DDS, 4:4 diaminodiphenyl sulphone)

Dapsone is still a most useful drug in the treatment of leprosy. It is a bacteriostatic agent and usually given in dosage of 6-10 mg/kg body weight per week. Side effects of dapsone are haemolytic anaemia, methaemoglobinaemia, agranulocytosis, psychosis, hepatitis and skin rash.

Rifampicin

It is a semisynthetic broad spectrum antibiotic which has a bactericidal effect against M. leprae. Varying dosage schedules have been tried but a monthly dose of 600 mg has proved to be as effective as daily doses and is less likely to evoke signs of toxicity. The common side effects are red discolouration of urine, abdominal pain, skin rash, thrombocytopaenia and 'flu' like syndrome.

Clofazimine

Clofazimine is iminophenazine dye which has a dual effect, bacteriostatic against M. leprae and anti-inflammatory against lepra reaction. It is given in dosage of 300-350 mg/week while in reactions, the dose being 300 mg daily. Side effects are red discolouration of urine, stool, sweat, sputum and tears and red brown pigmentation of skin and conjunctiva.

World Health Organization has recommended two therapeutic regimens, one for multibacillary leprosy (BB, BL, LL) and other for paucibacillary leprosy (TT, BT).

For paucibacillary leprosy: Rifampicin, 600 mg once monthly supervised and dapsone, 100 mg daily self administered. This treatment should be continued for a period of six months.

For multibacillary leprosy: Rifampicin, 600 mg once monthly supervised; Dapsone, 100 mg daily self administered; and clofazimine, 300 mg once monthly supervised. The treatment should be given at least

PLATE XIII

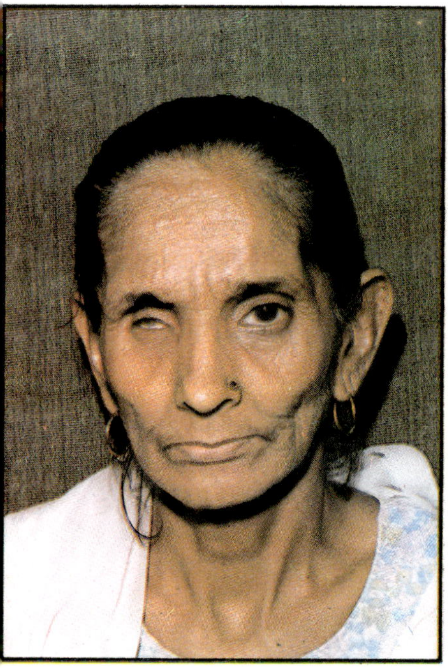

TUBERCULOID LEPROSY

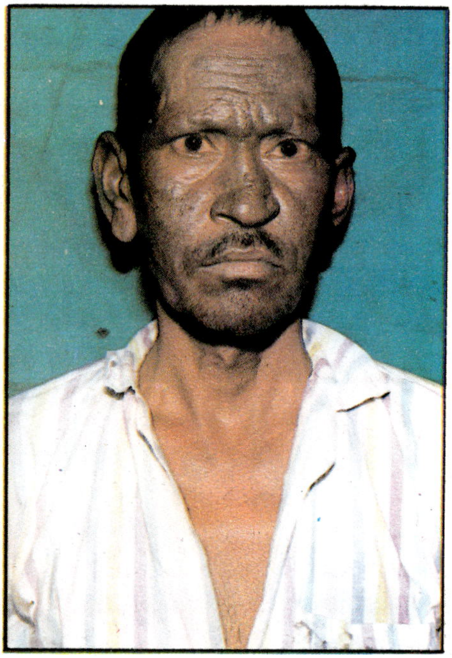

LEPROMATOUS LEPROSY

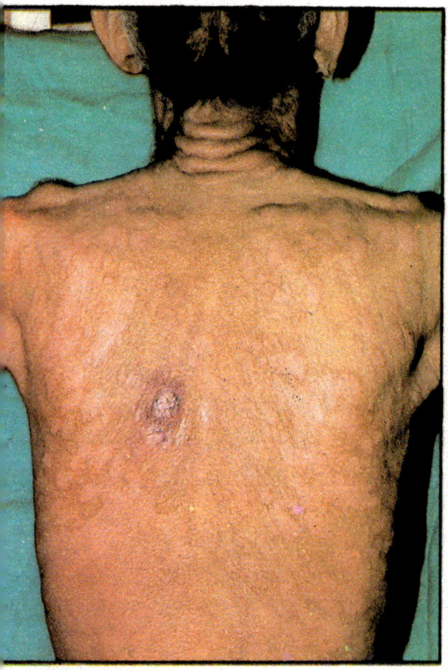

BORDERLINE LEPROMATOUS LEPROSY

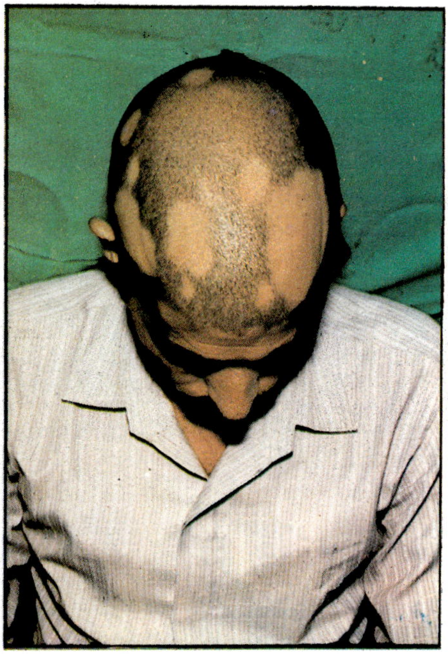

ALOPECIA AREATA

PLATE XIV

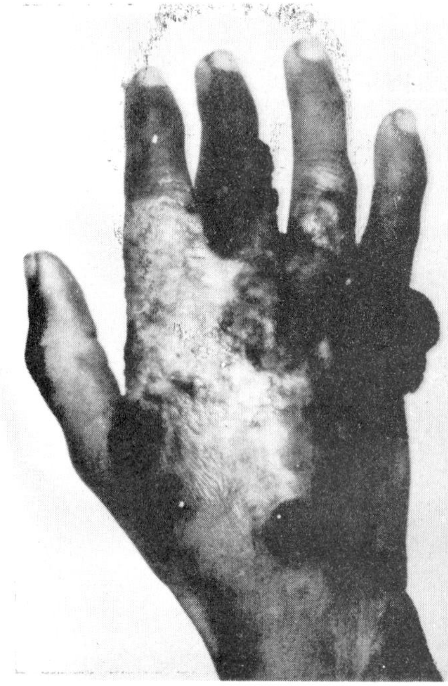

TUBERCULOSIS VERRUCOSA CUTIS

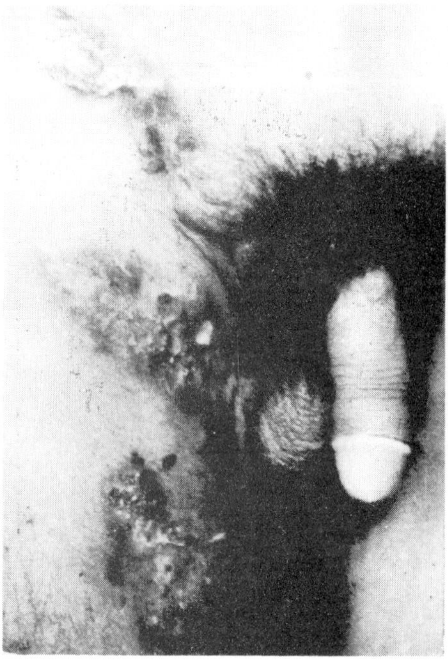

SCROFULODERMA

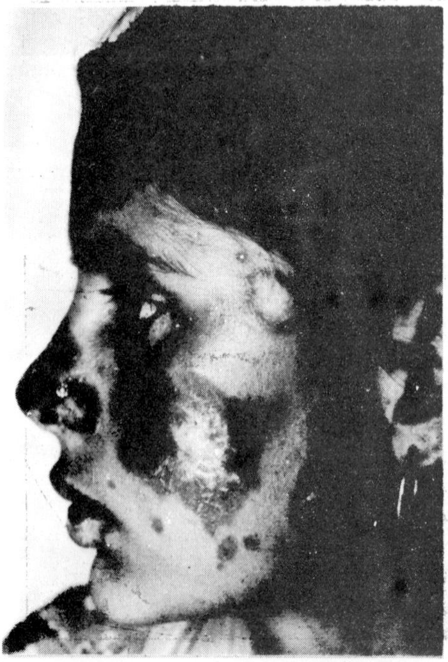

DISCOID LUPUS ERYTHEMATOSUS

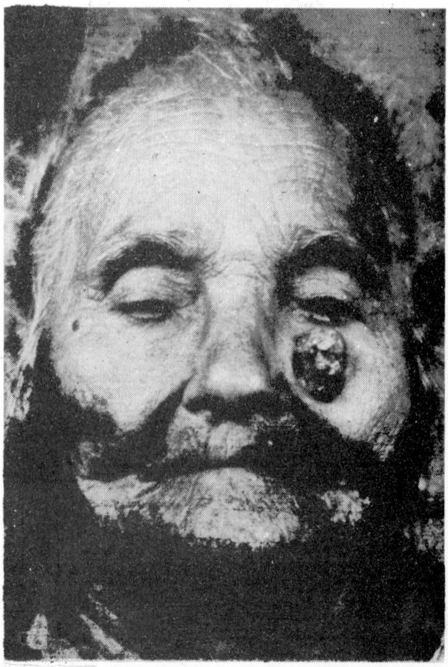

BASAL CELL CARCINOMA

PLATE XV

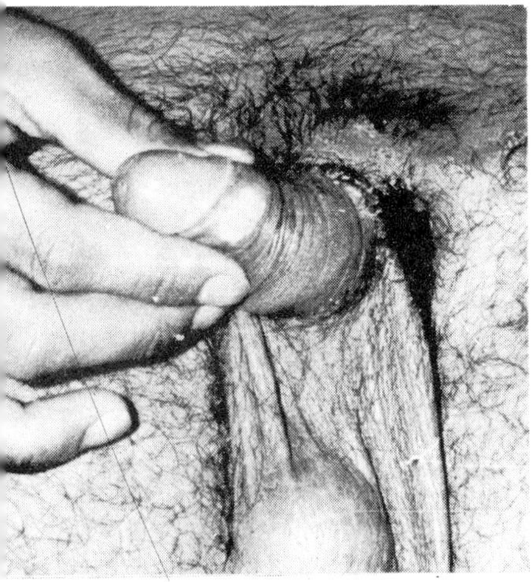

CHANCROID

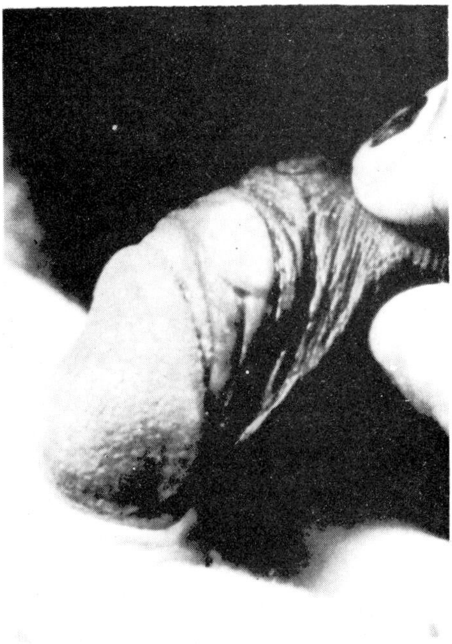

DONOVANOSIS

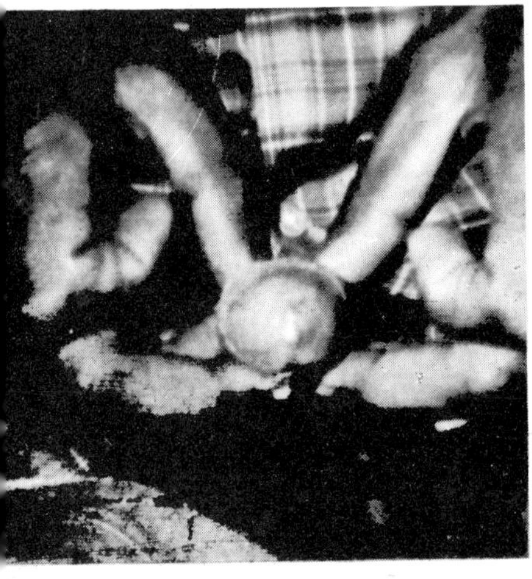

GONORRHEA

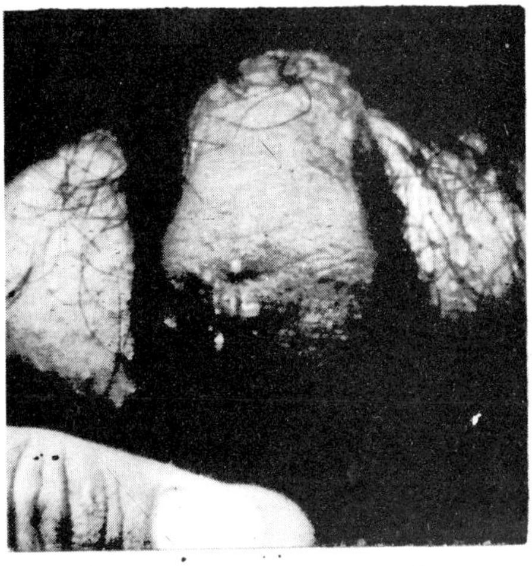

HERPES GENITALIS

PLATE XVI

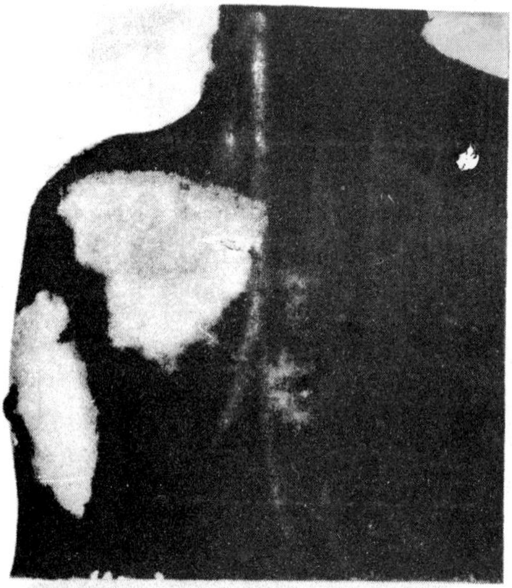

BORDERLINE TUBERCULOID LEPROSY

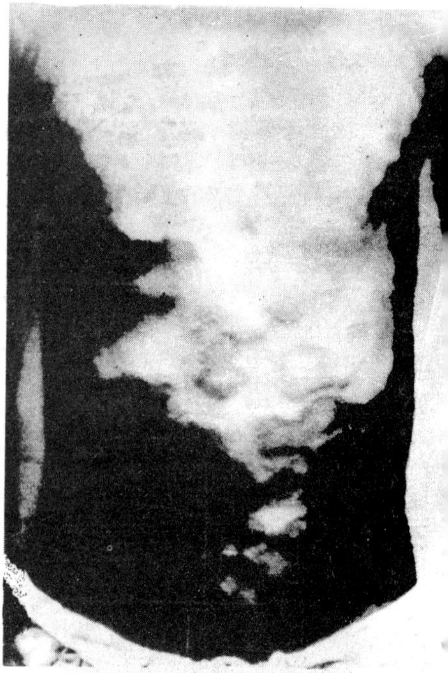

MID BORDERLINE LEPROSY

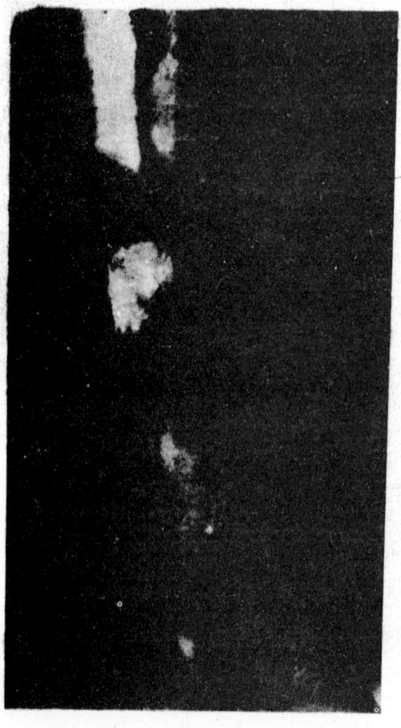

TUBERCULOID LEPROSY

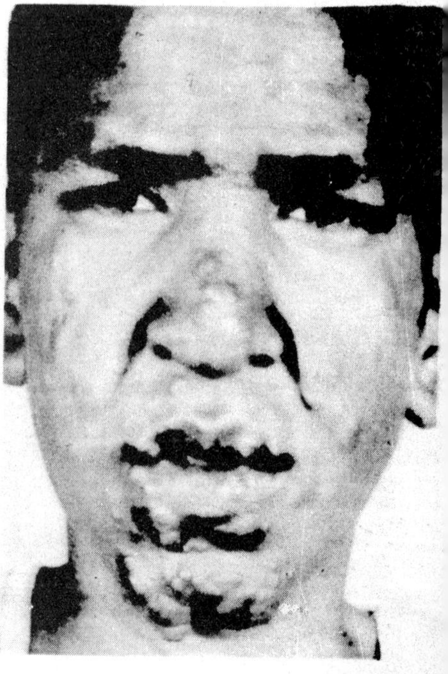

LEPROMATOUS LEPROSY

for a period of 2 years and be continued if possible upto smear negativity.

Treatment of Lepra Reactions

It is generally accepted that antileprosy drugs should not be discontinued during reaction phase. Treatment of reaction can be discussed under the two heads: specific measures and general measures.

Specific measures include certain specific antiinflammatory medications which are:

(a) corticosteroids, given in sufficient dosages (usually 30-40 mg) to control the acute reaction then tapering off as rapidly as possible.

(b) Clofazimine, given in dosage of 300 mg daily for 2-3 weeks, reducing to 200 mg daily for a month, and then to 100 mg daily. It is usually combined with steroids.

(c) Thalidomide, given in dosage of 300-400 mg per day in divided doses, gradually reducing by 100 mg a day every week. It is indicated only in patients with type II (ENL) reactions.

General measures include reassurance, physical and mental rest, removal of triggering factors, ingestion of appropriate analgesics and anti inflammatory agents, care of eyes and physiotherapy to prevent deformities.

Appendix

Common drugs for topical therapy:

Trade name	*Generic name*	*Concentration*
Soothing and antipruritic lotions		
Calamine lotion	Calamina	15 gm
(Boots)	Zinc oxide	0.5 gm
	Sodium citrate	500 mg
	Bentonite	3 gm
	Liq. Phenol	0.5 ml
	Glycerine	5 ml
Caladryl lotion	Calamina	8%
(Parke Davis)	Diphenhydramine HCl	1%
	Camphor	0.1%
	Denatured spirit	2.37%
Antibacterial preparations		
Betadine (Wockhardt)	Povidone iodine	5%
Neosporin (Burroughs-Wellcome)	Polymyxin B sulphate	5000 units
	Bacitracin zinc	400 units
	Neomycin sulphate	3400 units
Fucidin Leo (Carter Wallace)	Sod. Fusidate	2%
Soframycin (Roussel)	Framycetin sulphate	1%

Genticyn (Ind. Sch.)	Gentamycin sulphate	0.1%
Silver sulphadiazine (Indo-Pharma)	Silver Sulphadiazine	1%

Corticosteroid ointment and creams

Betnovate (Glaxo)	Betamethasone valerate	0.12%
Eumosone (Glaxo)	Clobetasone 17-butyrate	0.05%
Tenovate (Glaxo)	Clobetasone propionate	0.05%
Beclate (Cipla)	Beclomethasone dipropionate	0.25%
Flucort (Lyka)	Flucinolone acetonide	0.025%
Flucort H (Lyka)	Flucinolone acetonide	0.1%
Luci (Gufic)	Flucinolone acetonide	0.025%
Steriderm (Micro Lab)	Clobetasone 17-butyrate	0.05%
Steriderm-S (Micro Lab)	Clobetasone propionate	0.05%
Diprolene (Fulford)	Betamethasone dipropionate	0.64 mg/gm
Colsipan (Schering)	Flucortolone	1.25 mg
	Flucortolone caproate	1.25 mg

Corticosteroid ointments and cream with antibacterial agent

Betnovate-N (Glaxo)	Betamethasone valerate	0.025%
	Neomycin sulphate	0.5%
Beclate-N (Cipla)	Beclomethasone dipropionate	0.25%
	Neomycin sulphate	0.5%
Flucart-N (Lyka)	Flucinolone acetonide	0.025%
	Neomycin sulphate	0.5%
Diprogenta (Fulford)	Betamethasone dipropionate	0.64 mg/gm
	Gentamycin sulphate	1 mg/gm
Sofradex (Roussel)	Dexamethasone acetate	0.1%
	Fremycetin sulphate	1%
Genticyn HC (Ind. Schering)	Gentamycin sulphate	0.1%

Fucibet (Leo pharma)	Fusidic acid	20 mg/gm
	Betamethasone valerate	1.2 mg/gm
Colsipan-N (Schering)	Flucortolone caproate	0.5%
	Neomycin sulphate	0.33%

Antifungal ointments and creams

Micogel (Cipla)	Miconazole Nitrate	2%
Zole (Gufic)	Miconazole Nitrate	2%
Daktarin (Ethnor)	Miconazole Nitrate	2%
Tinaderm (Fuford)	Tolnaftate	1%
Lotril (Eclat)	Clotrimazole	1%
Surfaz (Franco-Indian)	Clotrimazole	1%
Canesten (Bayer)	Clotrimazale	1%

Antifungal ointments and cream with corticosteroids

Daktacort gel (Ethnor)	Miconazole Nitrate	2%
	Hydrocortisone acetate	1%
Micogel F (Cipla)	Miconazole nitrate	2%
Zole-F (Gufic)	Miconazole nitrate	2%
	Flucinolone acetonide	0.01%
Lotriderm (Fufford)	Clotrimazole	10 mg
	Betamethasone dipropionate	0.64 mg
Betnovate-C (Glaxo)	Chinoform	3%
	Betamethasone valerate	0.12%

Anticandidal agents

Mycostatin (Sarabai)	Nystatin	1,00,000 unit per gm
Natamycin (Martel Hammer)	Natamycin	2%
Surfaz (Franco Indian)	Clotrimazole	1%
Zole (Gufic)	Miconazole	2%
Micogel (Cipla)	Miconazole	2%
Inferina (Lyka)	Haymycin	0.5%

Anti scabies drugs

Ascabiol (May & Baker)	Benzyl Benzoate	25%
Crotorax (SG Pharma)	Crotamiton	10%
Emscab (MM Labs)	Gamma benzene hexachloride	1%
Gab lotion (Gufic)	Gamma benzene hexachloride	1%

Antipediculosis agent

Emscab (MM Labs)	Gamma benzene hexachloride	1%
Lorexane (ICI)	Gamma benzene haxachloride	1%
Gab lotion (Gufic)	Gamma benzene hexachloride	1%

Anti-acne preparations

Eudyna (German remedies)	Tretinoin	0.05%
Retino A (Ethnor)	Tretinoin	0.05%
Persol forte (Wallace)	Precipitated sulphur	5%
	Benzyl Peroxide	10%

Keratolytic and tar preparations

Cotaryl (FDC)	Urea	12%
	Calc. Lactate	0.5%
	Lactate	6%
	Pot. chloride	0.5%
	Mag. Chlor.	0.3%
	Aminoacetic acid (glycine)	3%
	Sod. Acid phos.	0.5%
	Amm. Chlo,	0.5%
	Sod. Chlor.	0.5%

Keralin (East India)	Benzoic acid	12%
	Salicylic acid	6%
	Hydrocortison acetate	0.5%
Derobin (Allenburys)	Dithranol	1.15%
	Salicylic acid	1.15%
	Sol. of Coal Tar	5.3%
Pragmatar (Eskay Lab.)	Cetyl alcohol	5%
	Cetyl tar distillate	4%
	Sulphur precipitated	3%
	Salicylic acid	3%
Sun screen preparation		
Paraminol (Griffon)	Para-amino benzoic acid	10%
Pabalak (Shalaks)	Para-amino-benzoic acid	5%

Index